Atlas of Pediatric Diseases

ATLAS
of
PEDIATRIC
DISEASES

DR. MED. HELMUT MOLL
Senior Medical Officer
Children's Unit, Maria Hospital Papenburg on Ems

Translated by
DR. MED. WALTER KLEINDIENST

1976
W. B. SAUNDERS COMPANY
Philadelphia · London · Toronto
GEORG THIEME PUBLISHERS
Stuttgart

Atlas of Pediatric Diseases

ISBN 0–7216–6430–X

Last digit is the print number: 9   8   7   6   5   4   3   2   1

Preface

"First of all, observe!"
(VIRCHOW 1862)

A disease with visible symptoms can often be better described by good illustrations than by long verbal elucidations. This is the reason for presenting this selection of pediatric pictures originating from my own department. The book emphasizes the visual aspects of pediatric affections as they are first seen in the clinic, at the bedside, or in the doctor's office. It is intended to serve the practitioner, the medical student, and the pediatric nurse as a practical guide toward the understanding of pediatric disease.

The accent here is on the illustrations, while the legends, consisting of concise case reports, are kept as brief as possible. The commentary on each disease follows a uniform systematic-nosological sequence of definition, etiology, and frequency, followed by data relating to clinical symptomatology and differential diagnosis. The sections on therapy are confined to a description of the principles of treatment.

All cases are personal observations except Fig. 114, which was kindly provided by *Professor David Smith* (Seattle). I hope this collection of pediatric pictures will confirm, complement, prepare for, or recall the reader's personal clinical experiences i.e., that it will teach to "watch and see," which will doubtless remain the basis of clinical diagnosis for many years to come in spite of data processing systems and computerized medicine.

I am deeply indebted to my colleagues at the clinic and to my medical and nursing personnel, without whose valuable aid I would hardly have accomplished this work in addition to my daily clinical routine. Special thanks are due to my chief resident Dr. ELISABETH KLESMANN and to Dr. GÜNTHER HAUFF and his colleagues of Georg Thieme Publishers. As always, the assistance of my wife and pediatric colleague Dr. HILDEGARD MOLL was decisive. This book, which during its preparation often interfered with our private life, is dedicated to her and to my children Christoph, Stephan, Martin, and Hildegard.

Papenburg, Spring 1975

HELMUT MOLL

Table of Contents

Atlas of Pediatric Diseases

Congenital Malformations

Down's Syndrome

Definition

Down's syndrome (formerly: mongolism or mongoloid idiocy) is a congenital malformation syndrome caused by chromosomal aberration with related mental retardation. Trisomy 21 (chromosome 21 in all trisomic instead of diploic cells, with a total chromosome set of 47 instead of 46) is characteristic in 94 per cent of all occurrences; in the remaining 6 per cent, about half are a "mosaic trisomy" (a trisomy 21 in only a portion of the somatic cells) and the other half are a "translocation trisomy" (additional chromosome 21 attached to another chromosome; a total set of 13 to 15 or 22 seemingly normal chromosomes). Trisomy 21 results from non-disjunction during meiosis. The frequency of the disease increases as the age of the mother advances. Beyond the age of 30 the rate doubles every five years. In the case of "translocation trisomy" there is no relation between incidence and maternal age. It is inherited from a phenotypically normal parent with a karyotype of 45 (balanced translocation) and rates at about 20 per cent among children of these parents. The morbidity rate of Down's syndrome per 1000 neonates is one to three cases.

Clinical Findings

1. Characteristic surface morphology includes: a mongoloid face with undifferentiated features; slanted palpebral fissures extending laterally from a deep medial origin, epicanthus (sickle-shaped skinfold above the inner angle of the eye); flat nasal bridge, open mouth with macroglossia of fissured tongue; brachycephalic head; dysplastic earlobes; laxity of skin, particularly of the neck; and white (Brushfield's) spots of the iris.

2. Retarded growth is evidenced by acromicria of the hands (distal shortening of the hand); clinodactyly (incurved little finger); brachymesophalangia of the fifth finger on X-ray; and a single transverse palmar crease. The distal axial triradius of the hypothenar is a typical skin pattern. Also characteristic is a wide space between first and second toes (sandal gap). Pelvic X-rays reveal reduced acetabular angles, wide but low ilia, and coxa valga.

3. Reduced muscle tone, frog belly and hyperextended joints are typical musculo-skeletal aberrations.

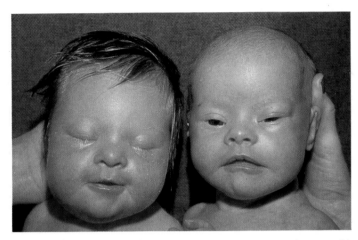

1   Different grades of mongoloid face in two newborns with trisomy 21.

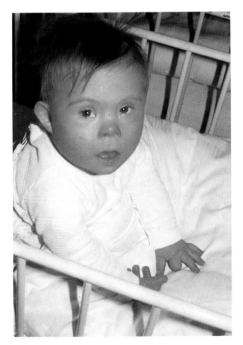

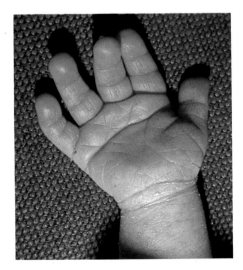

2   Eight-month-old infant with trisomy 21. Oblique palpebral fissures, epicanthus, retracted root of nose, open mouth, and undifferentiated earlobes are present. Age of mother: 43.

3   Simian line in Down's syndrome.

4. Mental retardation occurs in one of two types: the hypodynamic-oligophrenic type (good-natured, docile, loves music and may reach an IQ of 60), and the hyperdynamic-oligophrenic type (erethitic, moody, and seldom surpasses an IQ of 50).

Treatment   .

There is no specific therapy. Symptomatic improvement may be achieved by different pedagogic measures, physical exercises, and drugs.

Prognosis

Practical education proves beneficial. Antibiotics have decreased the former high mortality caused by low immunity. Acute leukemias occur more often in patients with Down's syndrome than in the general population.

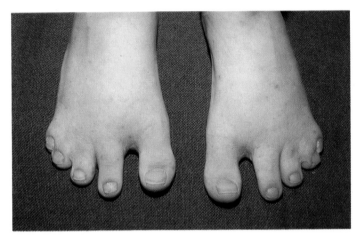

4   "Sandal gap" and syndactyly in Down's syndrome.

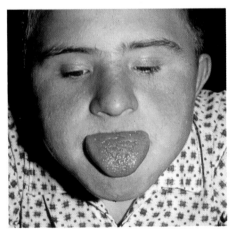

5   Scrotal or fissured tongue in Down's syndrome.

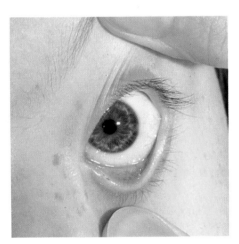

6   Brushfield's spots near the periphery of the iris are a frequent but unspecific finding in Down's syndrome.

Cleft Lip and Palate

Definition

The developmental defects in the lip and palatine region are either peristatic or are genetically determined in 15 to 30 per cent of the cases. The defects occur accordingly once among 500 neonates. Morphologically the following pictures are found:
1. Cleft upper lip: cheiloschisis, incomplete harelip.
2. Cleft of upper lip and alveolar process: cleft lip and palate, cheilognathoschisis, complete harelip.
3. Cleft of the soft and hard or soft palate: palatoschisis.
4. Cleft of lip, alveolar process, hard and soft palate: cheilognathopalatoschisis, total cleft. If bilateral, it is sometimes called "Wolf's jaws".

Clinical Findings

The functional disturbances relegate sucking and swallowing to feeding problems. Moreover, infections of the upper respiratory tract have an increased tendency. The development of speech is inhibited later.

Treatment

For the newborn and infant, tube-feeding may be necessary. Surgical treatment can be started from the fourth month. Clefts of lip and maxilla are closed in the first year, those of the soft palate in the second, and clefts of the hard palate in the fourth year.

Prognosis

With present-day maxillofacial techniques the prognosis is excellent regarding both cosmetic results and speaking abilities.

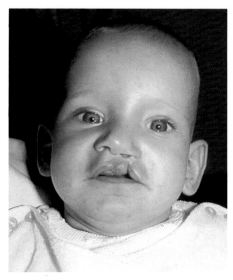

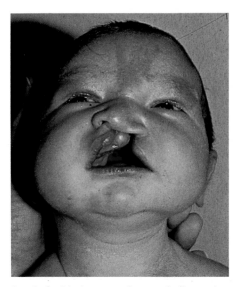

7   Hereditary left-sided partial cheilognathoschisis (with complete cleft palate) in a
six-month-old boy.

8   Left-sided complete cheilognathopalatoschisis in a newborn. Additional
finding: harmless nevus flammeus on
forehead and upper eyelids.

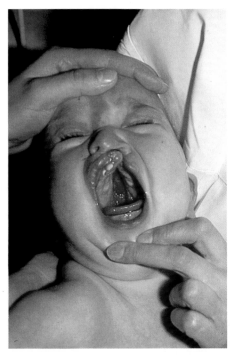

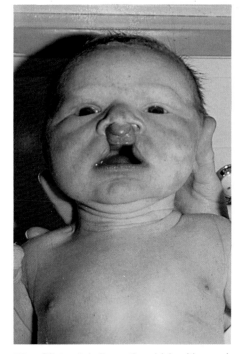

9   The infant in Fig. 8 at the age of six
months shortly before the first surgical
intervention. Dentition of the two right, upper
deciduous incisors has begun. The continuous complete cleft is visible.

10   Bilateral cheilognathoschisis with prominent os incisivum in a newborn. The same
malformation is present in one other of five
siblings.

Franceschetti's Syndrome

Definition

Franceschetti's syndrome (mandibulofacial dysostosis, Treacher-Collins syndrome) is a predominantly hereditary, but in most cases sporadically appearing malformation of varying manifestations in the facial area. Both bones and soft tissues arising from the first branchial arch and cleft are affected.

Clinical Findings

Typical morphological features are:
1. Antimongoloid palpebral fissures, a split lateral portion of the lower lid and, in rarer cases, of the upper lid (coloboma of the eyelids).
2. Mandibular, maxillary, and jugular hypoplasia (bird face), macrostomia with anomalies of dental position and occlusion (fish-mouth physiognomy).
3. Low-set ears with dysplastic earlobes, atresia of the auditory meatus.

Differential Diagnosis

1. Craniofacial dysostosis (Crouzon's disease)
2. Acrocephalosyndactyly (Apert's syndrome)
3. Rubinstein's syndrome
4. Cornelia de Lange syndrome
5. Pierre Robin syndrome (See p. 10)
6. Bonnevie-Ullrich-Turner syndrome
7. Hurler-Pfaundler's syndrome (dysostosis multiplex)

Treatment

Plastic surgery is feasible after infancy (blepharoplasty, otoplasty).

Prognosis

The syndrome does not progress nor does it affect the brain. Malformations of the middle and inner ear are rare.

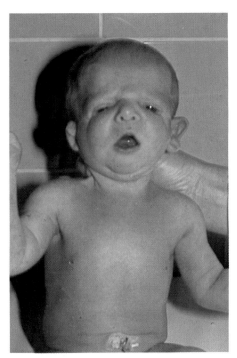

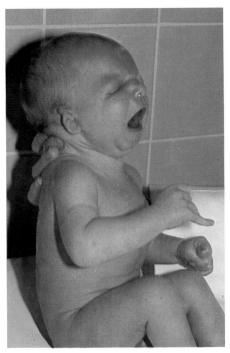

11 Franceschetti's syndrome in a six-day-old boy. Note how the position of eyes differs from mongolism. Macrostomia is also characteristic.

12 Mandibular hypoplasia with receding chin. Low, hypoplastic auricle with atresia of the auditory canal is typical.

Pierre Robin Syndrome

Definition

The Pierre Robin syndrome is a malformation simultaneously affecting the mandibular and glossal area. It is hereditary and most probably a genetic defect consisting of the following triad: microgenia (mandibular hypoplasia), glossoptosis (tongue falling backwards), and cleft palate.

Clinical Findings

Respiratory and nutritional distress may result from mandibular hypoplasia, which appears in the newborn as a receding lower jaw, as well as from the tongue falling backwards into the cleft palate. The functional manifestations are dominated by dyspnea with inspiratory stridor, apneic-cyanotic attacks, or problems with drinking. Suffocation, hypoxemic brain damage, and aspiration pneumonia are threatening complications.

Differential Diagnosis

Franceschetti's syndrome (See p. 8.)

Treatment

As immediate measures the patient should be placed in a prone position. If necessary, pull the tongue forward with a tongue forceps. Use a permanent gastric tube for feeding. Life-threatening respiratory disturbances will in most cases disappear spontaneously, and mandibular growth will increase over several months of conservative treatment. Only in rare cases will operative extension of the mandible and fixation of the tongue with nylon sutures be required. Correction of the cleft palate can be done during the second to fourth year in the usual way.

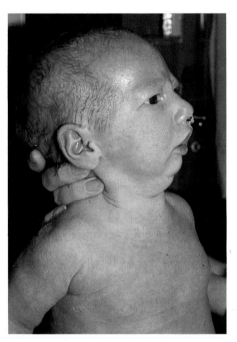

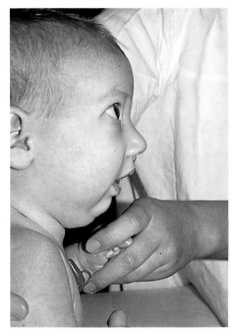

13 Robin's syndrome in a four-week-old girl. Receding lower jaw, double chin, stridor and cyanosis in the recumbent position, and inability to drink are noted.

14 Functional improvement following conservative treatment at the age of three months. After seven months, the microgenia is largely compensated.

Klippel-Feil Syndrome

Definition

The so-called short-neck syndrome is a dominant hereditary trait which results from an inhibited differentiation of the cervical spine before the third month of embryonic life. This results in fusion of cervical vertebrae into solid osseous masses.

Clinical Findings

The head appears to arise directly from the body (frog neck), lateral movement of the head is limited. The hair line is low on the neck. Fissures, synostoses and hypoplastic deformities of the cervical vertebrae bodies appear on roentgenograms. In addition, a variety of other malformations may be present.

Treatment

There is no treatment.

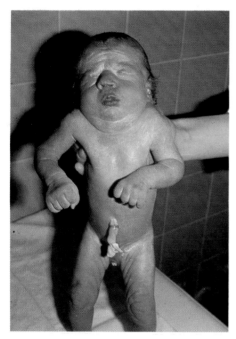

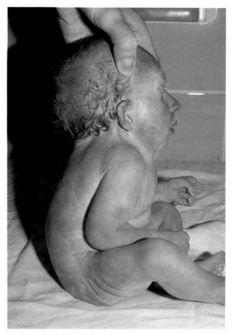

15 Premature infant with Klippel-Feil syndrome. The head seems to rest between the shoulders owing to compressed cervical vertebrae. Median cleft palate is an additional malformation.

16 A thick frog-like neck, low border of back hair, and impossible lateral movement of the head are characteristic.

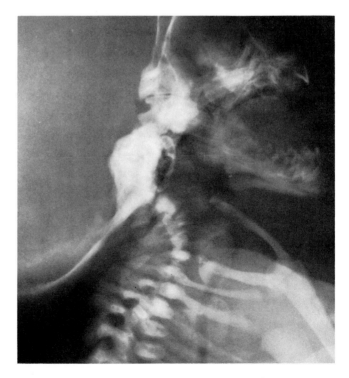

17 A coherent mass of cervical vertebrae that is impossible to differentiate on roentgenograms.

Coccygeal Teratoma

Definition

Coccygeal teratomas are congenital tumors containing portions of all three germinal layers in different grades of differentiation. In the case of high differentiation of the tissue (adult teratoma) malformations are most prominent. In immature forms (embryonic teratoma) the tumorous character tends toward malignancy. The malignancy rate is between ten and twenty percent. The incidence in girls is five times as high as in boys.

Clinical Findings

The spheric, sometimes monstrous tumors, which may impede delivery, arise with a broad base from the coccyx. The anus and rectum are displaced anteriorly. The consistency of the tumors ranges from firm to elastic. In about 40 per cent of the patients, calcifications are seen on roentgenograms. In malignant degeneration, which becomes increasingly threatening after the fourth month of life, pulmonary and skeletal metastases may be found.

Treatment

Radical extirpation between the second and the fourth week of life is the preferred method of treatment.

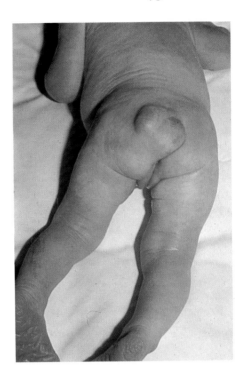

18   Newborn girl with a coccygeal teratoma the size of an egg.

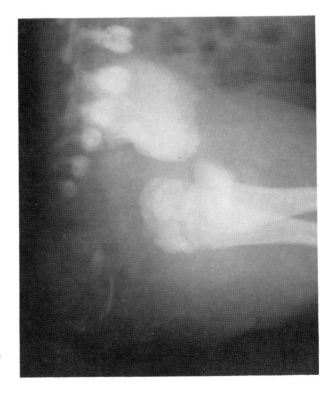

19   Clasp-like calcification within the teratoma visible on roentgenograms. Extirpation was made at the age of five weeks. No histologic signs of malignancy are present.

Diabetic Embryopathy and Fetopathy

Definition

Diabetic embryopathy is characterized by organic malfomations which occur within the first ten weeks of pregnancy in children of diabetic mothers. The incidence is about 5 to 10 per cent, perhaps increasing with the duration and severity of maternal diabetes and particularly diabetic angiopathy. Diabetic fetopathy arises after the third month of pregnancy. Fetal death, abortion, macrosomia or postnatal disturbances of adaptation may result. The degree of the disorder depends greatly on the management of maternal diabetes during pregnancy. The mortality in infants of diabetic mothers ranges from 10 to 15 per cent.

Clinical Findings

Diabetic embryopathy is manifested by a broad spectrum of malformations: agenesis of different skeletal portions of the lower body, skeletal dysplasia (caudal regression), situs inversus and congenital heart defects. Infants with diabetic fetopathy are born prematurely, but they are overweight and oversize (macrosomia, giant babies, birth weight exceeding 4500 g, cushingoid appearance). Neonatal hypoglycemia caused by islet cell hyperplasia, increased postnatal jaundice and erythroblastosis are frequent findings. The infants are susceptible to cyanosis, the respiratory distress syndrome, thrombosis of renal veins, and infections. The mortality is 10 to 30 per cent.

Prevention

To prevent diabetic fetopathy, optimal management of maternal diabetes is necessary as well as induced premature delivery between the 36th and 38th week of pregnancy.

Treatment

Newborns with diabetic fetopathy are treated as premature infants.

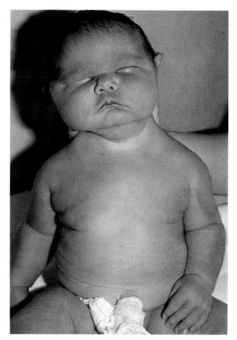

20   Giant baby of diabetic mother. Spontaneous delivery occurred three weeks before the estimated term. Weight: 5380 g; length: 59 cm. Congenital heart disease was present.

Traumatic Birth

Facial Palsy

Definition

Facial palsy after delivery involves injury to the peripheral portion of the seventh cranial nerve by pressure from a forceps blade or a pelvic bone distal to the stylomastoid foramen. Aside from brachial, palsy, it is the most common paresis post partum. The general incidence, including all minor forms, is about 6 per cent.

Clinical Findings

When the infant cries, the affected corner of the mouth does not move, the nasolabial fold is flat, the eyelids of the affected side are closed incompletely, and there is no wrinkling of the forehead. In the majority of cases, paresis is unilateral, with the lower branch of the nerve mostly affected.

Differential Diagnosis

Central facial paralysis, which results from intranatal hemorrhage into the supranuclear tract between the cerebral cortex and the pons, causes contralateral insufficiency of labial and buccal muscles (lower and medial branch). The innervation of the frontal and palpebral muscles (upper branch) remains intact. The peripheral type of congenital facial palsy (paralysis of all three branches) caused by nuclear aplasia (Moebius) is often combined with aplasia of other nuclei of cranial nerves, especially of the abducens nerve. This type shows no tendency to regress.

Treatment

Treatment is not necessary. Spontaneous healing occurs within a few weeks.

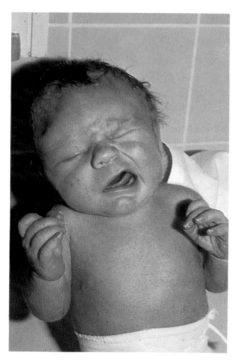

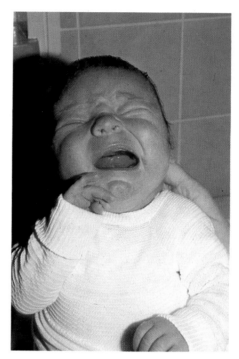

21   Newborn with right-sided facial palsy after forceps delivery. Depression of the skull (molding) over the right frontal bone was caused by a forceps blade. No neurologic signs are evident.

22   Restitution is almost complete after seven days.

Brachial Plexus Palsy

Definition

Brachial plexus palsy (Erb-Duchenne paralysis) is the most common postpartum paralysis. It is caused by intranatal tearing or compression of the roots of the fifth or sixth cervical nerves (cranial portion of the cervical plexus) resulting in flaccid paralysis of shoulder and upper arm. Overweight infants and those delivered from breech presentation or by forceps are predisposed.

Clinical Findings

The arm is extended and adducted (paralysis of deltoid, biceps and brachialis muscles), internally rotated (infraspinatus and teres minor muscles) and pronated (biceps and supinator muscles). Active elevation of the arm and flexion of the elbow are impossible. Flexion of hand and fingers is not affected. Frequent simultaneous involvement of the fourth cervical segment causes paralysis of the diaphragm (Kofferath syndrome).

Differential Diagnosis

1. Paralysis of the lower brachial plexus (nerves originating from C 8 and T 1, Klumpke's paralysis) is less common and the prognosis is less favorable. Neither the hand nor the fingers can be moved in this case. Position of the arm resembles that of Erb-Duchenne paralysis since in almost all cases the cranial roots are also affected slightly. If the sympathetic portion of the first thoracic nerve is involved, Horner's syndrome will appear (miosis, ptosis, apparent enophthalmos).

2. Epiphysiolysis of the humeral head.

3. Humeral fracture.

4. Clavicular fracture.

5. Parrot's pseudoparalysis in congenital syphilis.

Treatment

To attain immobilization and to prevent contractures, treatment consists of splinting the abducted and externally rotated upper arm with the forearm flexed (Spitzy). Massage and passive exercises should not be started until the third week.

Prognosis

Prognosis is favorable in most cases. Complete restoration may take three to six months. Muscular weakness, particularly in the deltoid, may persist.

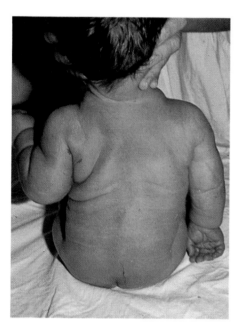

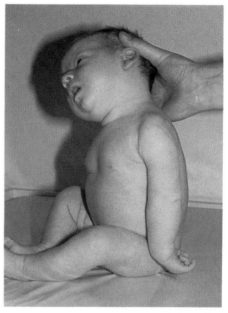

23 Right-sided upper brachial plexus palsy after difficult delivery of an infant weighing 5100 g. Adduction with internal rotation and pronation of the paralyzed arm are corresponding signs.

24 Erb-Duchenne paralysis in four-week-old infant weighing 4100 g at birth. The arm is hanging down in a typical position with adduction, internal rotation and pronation. Complete restitution within six months.

Cerebral Hemorrhage

Definition

Several factors are responsible for most cases of cerebral hemorrhage during delivery. Trauma, disturbed venous return owing to negative pressure with the emerging head, hypoxemia, hemorrhagic diathesis and increased capillary fragility of the newborn are among the major causative factors. In the total number of intracranial hemorrhages during delivery, hypoxemia is a much more common cause than mechanical injury by a ratio of 50 to 80 per cent versus 20 per cent.

Mechanical trauma (large babies, breech presentation, forceps) causes laceration of the dura with subsequent subdural hematoma. When there is laceration of the falx and hemorrhage from the superior sagittal sinus, the hematoma is found supratentorially on the frontal and parietal convexities. If the tentorium or the straight or transverse sinuses are ruptured, the hematoma lies supra or infratentorially. *Stasis and hypoxemia* are often responsible for petechial diapedetic intracerebral hemorrhage into the parenchyma of the cerebral medulla. These may also cause bleeding by rhexis into the lateral ventricles and the basal nuclei in the area of the V. cerebri magna (Galeni) and the area of its afferent blood vessels (V. thalamostriata or terminalis). Asphyctic and premature newborns are predilected. Leptomeningeal hemorrhage (subarachnoidal hemorrhage) into the parieto-occipital convexity takes up an intermediate position both pathogenetically and topographically; it may be caused by trauma or hypoxia.

Clinical Findings

The symptoms of cerebral hemorrhage in the newborn correspond to the manifold possibilities of central irritation or paralysis: apathy, hypotension, less frequently hypertension (often different on the two sides), yawning, "cri encéphalique", pale cyanosis, central dyspnea, disturbances of temperature regulation with hyper- or hypothermia, nystagmus, anisocoria, visual paralyses and focal convulsions. Bulging fontanel and sanguinolent or xanthochromic cerebrospinal fluid may be present. External signs of traumatic delivery, such as forceps marks, cephalhematoma, bleeding from ear and nose, facial palsy or fracture of the skull, may indicate intracranial hemorrhage.

Differential Diagnosis

Clinically it is often impossible to differentiate cerebral hemorrhage from asphyxia and the respiratory distress syndrome.

Treatment

The most essential measures for treatment are immobilization, keeping the infant warm and well oxygenated in the incubator, tube-feeding and hemostatic treatment. Subdural hematoma is aspirated by puncture of the fontanel.

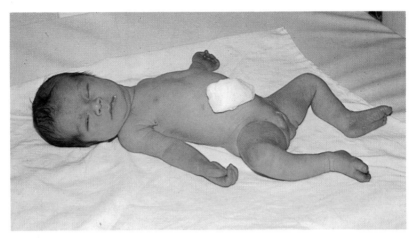

25 Eight-hour-old newborn with cerebral hemorrhage owing to traumatic birth. Complicated delivery occurred after transverse presentation and podalic version. Pallor, somnolence, cerebral facies, a temperature of 33.9°C and a slightly bulging fontanel are present.

Prognosis

Prognosis depends on localization and extent of hemorrhage. In cases with clinically relevant symptoms, mortality is high and long-term prognosis poor.

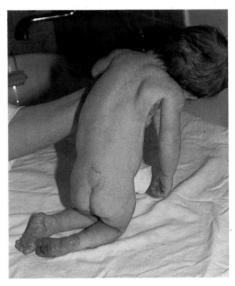

26 Striking muscular hypotonia.

Facial Hemorrhage

Definition

Petechial cutaneous hemorrhage in the face of the newborn is a result of the combined effect of three factors: disturbed venous return, hypoxemia, and hemorrhagic diathesis. But often it will not be possible to decide which of the factors plays the leading causative role. Intrauterine hypoxemia and hypoxemia during delivery which cause injury to the capillary endothelium are of major importance. Physiologic diminution of clotting factors VII, IX, X and prothrombin in the neonatal period are of lesser importance as a primary cause of hemorrhage. Prematurity is an additional detrimental factor.

Clinical Findings

Slight facial and acrocyanosis of the healthy newborn immediately after delivery is caused by low oxygen content of the blood about 4 vol per cent (normal 20 vol per cent in arterial and 12 vol per cent in venous blood). Together with the corresponding high CO_2 content, this stimulates the respiratory center. Compression of the thorax during delivery and the resulting disturbance of venous return may cause deeper local cyanosis of the face with multiple petechiae, even subconjunctival hemorrhage.

Differential Diagnosis

Cyanosis and hemorrhage caused by congestion may simulate blue asphyxia. Normal dermal circulation in the remaining parts of the body, and normal vitality and normal blood gas analysis exclude the above. Although cutaneous and mucosal hemorrhage of the face are usually harmless, cerebral hemorrhage must be considered if these manifestations are evident.

Treatment

Uncomplicated facial hemorrhage is absorbed spontaneously within one to four weeks. Thus, treatment is not necessary.

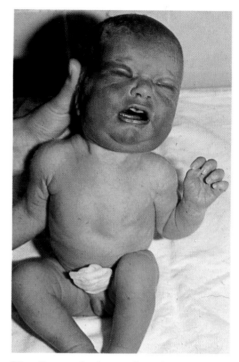

27   Congestive hemorrhage in the face of a viable newborn. Second day of life.

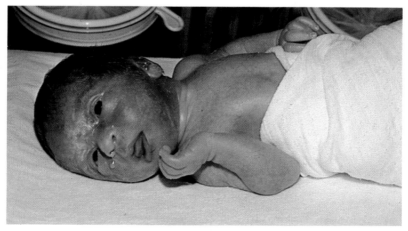

28   Premature infant weighing 1500 g with extensive facial hemorrhage. After cesarean section and a brief blue asphyxia (anesthesia) the trunk and extremities were pink. Death from ventricular hemorrhage occurred six hours later.

Cephalhematoma Resulting from Face Presentation

Definition

Cephalhematoma, called caput succedaneum in vertex presentation, is caused
by negative pressure and disturbed reflux of
blood and lymph while the head emerges.

Clinical Findings

The pasty, edematous soft-tissue swelling
shows petechial hemorrhage and, in vertex
presentation, affects the scalp. Bluish-
black, hemorrhagic discoloration of the skin
is a striking feature (circumocular hematoma, subconjunctival hemorrhage) in face
presentation, and hematoma of the buttocks in breech presentation.

Differential Diagnosis

Cephalhematoma is differentiated from
caput succedaneum by the fact that in the
latter the hematoma is not limited by suture
lines (See p. 30.).

Treatment

Treatment is not necessary. Cephalhematoma disappears spontaneously within the
first two days of life. Cutaneous and subcon-
two days of life. Cutaneous and subconjunctival hemorrhages are absorbed within
a few weeks.

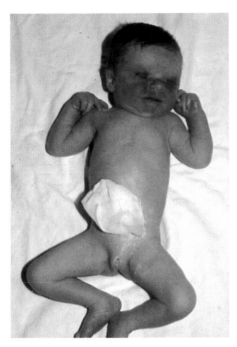

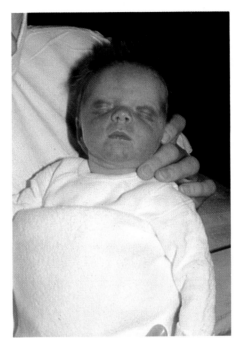

29   Facial hemorrhage in a viable premature infant (2220 g) after delivery by face
presentation. First day of life.

30   Twelfth day of life. Bilateral circumocular hematoma has not yet been absorbed.
The infant is clinically healthy.

Cephalhematoma after Vacuum Extraction

Definition

Vaccum extraction, initiated by Malmström in 1954, has largely replaced forceps in Scandinavia and Germany. The negative pressure of 0.6 to 0.9 kg/cm² on the head of the infant produces an artificial caput succedaneum.

Clinical Findings

Artificial cephalhematoma appears markedly circumscribed. Sliding off the vacuum extractor or continuous traction for more than 30 minutes may cause larger excoriation of the scalp.

Prognosis

The tendency to disappear spontaneously is the same as with natural caput succedaneum. Cutaneous injuries will heal quickly under aseptic conditions. The risk of intracranial damage appears equal to that of spontaneous labor, but lower than in forceps delivery.

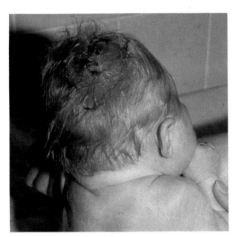

31   Scalp injury of a newborn caused by a vacuum extractor.

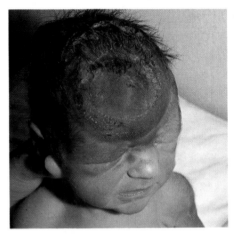

32 a   Cephalhematoma of scalp and forehead 6 hours after vacuum extraction from vertex presentation.

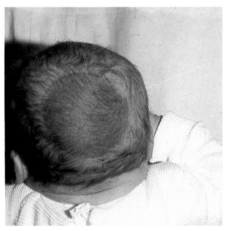

32 b   Suction cup suffusion of the scalp twelve hours after delivery.

Cephalhematoma

Definition

Cephalhematoma is a subperiosteal hematoma of the skull. It occurs when the mechanics of childbirth cause separation of the exterior periosteum and laceration of subperiosteal blood vessels. The incidence is 0.5 per cent of all newborns; it is higher among firstborns and in difficult deliveries.

Clinical Findings

The fluctuant, painless swelling becomes evident on the second day of life. The right parietal bone is the preferred site. During the first week it may increase from the size of a nut to that of an apple. It disappears between the 4th and 12th week. In the periphery an osseous wall can be palpated. Parchment-like crepitation is felt on top of the hematoma owing to lamellar ossification of the separated periosteum. Simul-taneous fracture of the skull is found in 25 per cent of newborns with cephalhematoma, and intracranial hematoma is found in 0.5 per cent.

Differential Diagnosis

Cephalhematoma is limited to one cranial bone. In contrast to *caput succedaneum* it does not cross suture lines. *Encephalocele* is always located around suture lines of fontanels.

Treatment

Heparin-containing ointments aid absorption. In exceptional cases aseptic puncture and antibiotic protection may be required. Infection and phlegmon of the scalp would be the most severe complications after puncture.

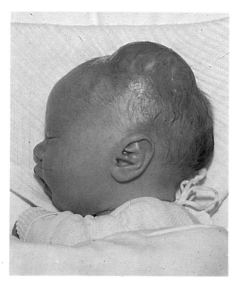

33 Cephalhematoma over the left parietal bone in a firstborn after breech presentation. Fifth day of life.

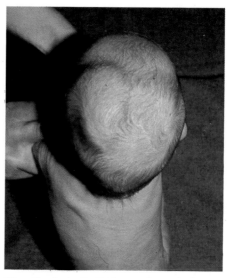

34 Typical limitation of cephalhematoma by clearly visible coronal, sagittal and lambdoid sutures.

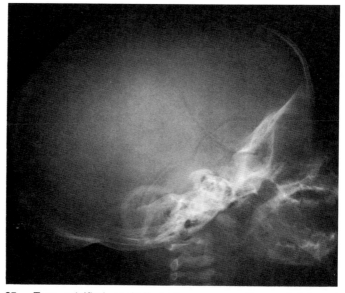

35 Two calcified cephalhematomas over the occipital and posterior parietal bones in a 10-week-old infant.

Forceps Mark

Definition

Forceps marks are pressure marks in the skin of the head of a newborn. Narrow pelvis, osseous prominences (promontory, symphysis) may cause similar marks, even on spontaneous delivery.

Clinical Findings

There are red, ecchymotic striae or spots, most frequently found over parietal and temporal bones and on cheeks. Necroses are rare findings.

Differential Diagnosis

Rare congenital circumscript skin defects may resemble necrotic pressure marks.

Treatment

Sterile dressing is sufficient.

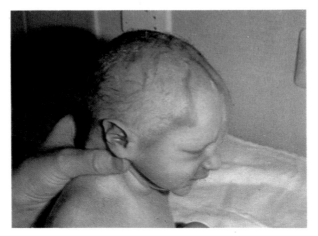

36   Typical streaklike pressure mark after forceps delivery, one hour post partum.

Congenital Compression of the Skull

Definition

Abnormal intrauterine position or pressure by promontory or forceps may cause impressions (pingpong-ball impression, molding) in the elastic skull of the infant without proof of fracture on roentgenograms.

Clinical Findings

The spoonlike or round impression is most frequently found on the parietal bone, less frequently on frontal and temporal bones. There are no neurologic symptoms. If central nervous irritation is present, depressed fracture with cerebral contusion and intracranial hematoma must be considered.

Treatment

Pingpong-ball impressions disappear spontaneously or may quite simply be corrected by means of an obstetrical vacuum extractor (largest cup, lowest vacuum). Surgical intervention is not necessary.

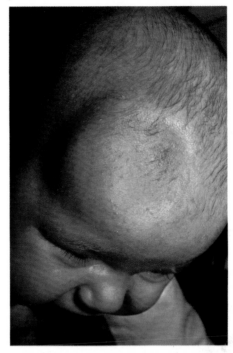

37   Four-week-old infant with congenital impression of the right temporal bone. No fracture. No neurologic symptoms. Spontaneous correction within the first six months.

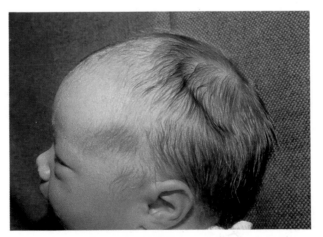

38   Molding of the left parietal bone of a newborn after delivery by the inverted Prague maneuver.

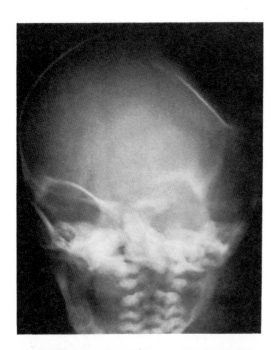

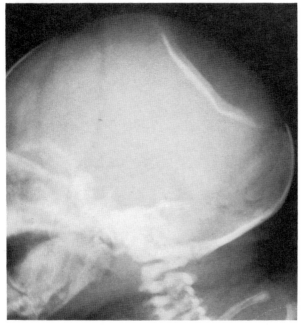

39 a and b   Deep depression on roentgenogram; fracture uncertain.

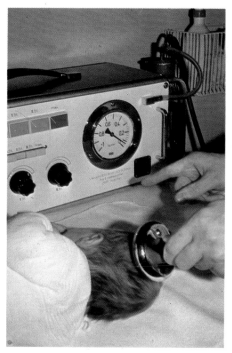

40   Lifting of ping-pong ball depression by means of vacuum extractor (diameter of suction cup 6 cm, negative pressure 0.2 kg/cm^2).

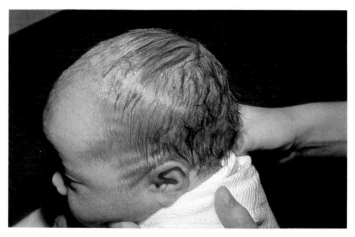

41   Normal clinical findings immediately after reposition of cranial depression. NAD on roentgenograms.

Fracture of Clavicle

Definition

Fracture of the clavicle is the most frequent bone injury to the infant during delivery. Greenstick fracture or, less frequently, complete fracture happens with presentation of the anterior shoulder of heavy or large infants.

Clinical Findings

Often the fracture causes no symptoms and will therefore be overlooked, or sometimes it is not evident until a week after delivery when marked callus formation indicates the disorder. Sometimes the arm is moved cautiously and hangs down in slight interior rotation. Palpation of the clavicle is painful; in complete fracture crepitation is present.

Differential Diagnosis

Erb-Duchenne paralysis (brachial plexus palsy — See p. 20.)

Treatment

Incomplete fracture requires no immobilization. With complete fracture, fixation of the arm to the trunk in cubital flexion (Desault's bandage) for two weeks will be sufficient. No functional disturbances will remain after healing of the fracture.

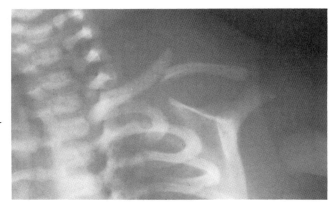

42   Left-sided complete fracture of clavicle in newborn of 4000 g. Typical site of fracture in the middle third and displacement of the medial fragment in cranio-posterior direction.

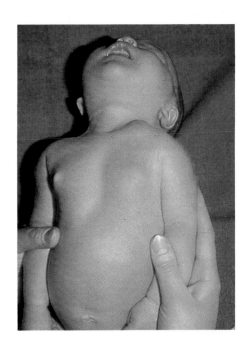

43   Clinical findings of the twelfth day of life: visible and palpable callus. No crepitation.

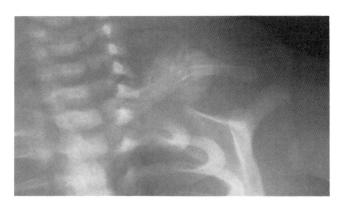

44   Fracture firmly consolidated three weeks after delivery. Solid, globular callus is apparent on roentgenograms.

Fracture of Humerus

Definition

Fracture of the humerus is usually caused by difficult delivery during breech presentation or cesarean section. The most common type is diaphyseal fracture. Epiphyseolysis of the head of the humerus is far less common.

Clinical Findings

Because of the painful state, the arm hangs down in flaccid pseudoparalysis. Palpation causes pain and crepitation. In *epiphyseolysis,* pseudoparalysis and internal rotation of the arm are present, soon followed by swelling of the shoulder. Since the head of the humerus is cartilaginous, roentgenologic diagnosis of dislocation is difficult, but becomes evident after a week when callus forms.

Differential Diagnosis

1. Fracture of clavicle (See p. 38.)
2. Erb-Duchenne paralysis
   (brachial plexus palsy-See p. 20.)
3. Parrot's pseudoparalysis

Treatment

Diaphyseal fracture of the humerus is treated by anchoring the arm to the trunk with the elbow flexed (Desault's bandage) for two weeks. *Epiphyseolysis* of the head of the humerus demands that the arm be immobilized by a dorsal splint with abduction of the shoulder joint and rectangular flexion of the elbow (Spitzy splint).

Prognosis

Like all other fractures in the newborn, humeral fracture will consolidate after two weeks under massive callus formation. Even severe dislocations will be corrected completely.

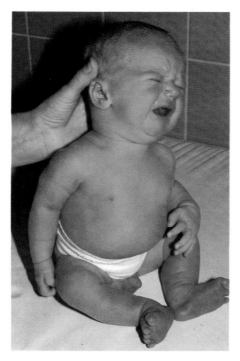

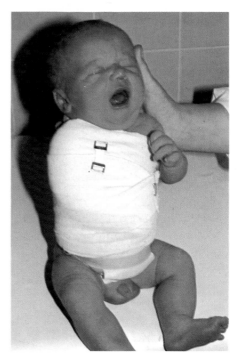

45 Right-sided diaphyseal fracture of humerus in a newborn after breech delivery. Pseudoparalysis, shortening and swelling of the humerus, and crepitation occurred.

46 Immobilization with a modified Desault's bandage.

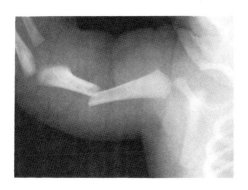

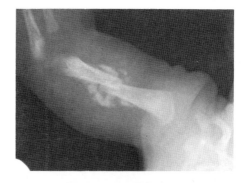

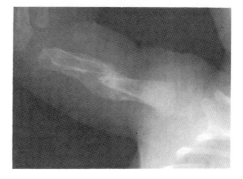

47 Complete diaphyseal fracture with axial and longitudinal displacement of fragments. First day of life.

48 Solid, bullet-like callus after two weeks.

49 Spontaneous correction of axial and longitudinal displacement after six weeks.

Epiphyseolysis of the Femoral Head

Definition

Epiphyseolysis of the proximal femoral epiphysis in traumatic birth is a fracture of the completely cartilaginous femoral neck. Like diaphyseal femoral fracture, it is usually caused by pulling the infant's leg during breech extraction.

hematoma and subsequent callus formation. In the beginning, only the latero-cranial displacement of the femur can be seen on roentgenograms, because the femoral head is still cartilaginous and not radiopaque. A similar picture is seen in congenital dislocation of the hip. Massive callus formation becomes evident after a week.

Clinical Findings

The first signs are reflex immobilization of the affected leg and pain on passive movement. Later, there are shortening of the leg, external rotation and swelling of the trochanteric area caused by subperiosteal

Treatment

A favorable prognosis is promised by immobilization in marked abduction and slight internal rotation (molded cast) or extension utilizing adhesive strapping over a period of two to three weeks.

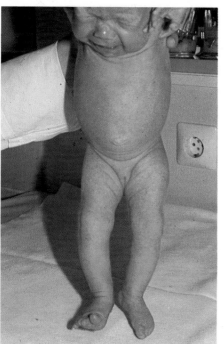

50 Epiphysiolysis of the left femoral head owing to difficult delivery. Swelling occurred over the left lateral, proximal portion of the femur with shortening of the leg, external rotation and pain. Three weeks after delivery.

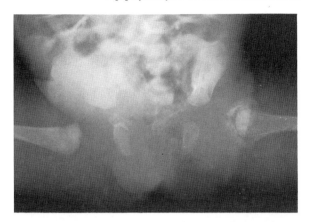

51   Mushroomlike callus and calcifying subperiosteal hemorrhage on roentgenograms. Three weeks after delivery.

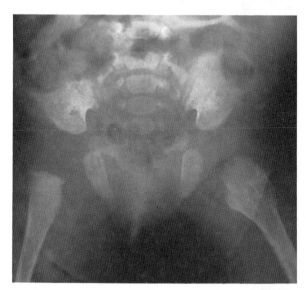

52   Club-shaped thickening of femoral neck seven weeks after delivery.

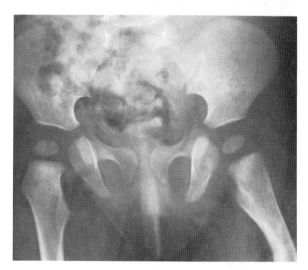

53   Normal morphology and function at the age of 11 months.

Pathology of the Newborn Infant

Erythema Toxicum Neonatorum

Definition

Erythema toxicum neonatorum is an allergic exanthem of variable appearance, intensity and duration in the first two weeks of life. This clinically benign disorder was first described by Leiner in 1912, who called it toxic erythema. The synonoms, exanthema allergicum neonatorum, urticaria neonatorum and possibly bullosis allergica are more precise. With the more transient forms included, it appears in about 50 per cent of all newborns.

Clinical Findings

Morbilliform, confluent, urticarial or, less frequently, small vesicular efflorescences are spread over the trunk and extremities and rarely last more than a few days. Localization and intensity undergo rapid change. In many cases vasomotor disturbance, red or white dermography or factitious urticaria are present. There is blood and tissue eosinophilia.

Differential Diagnosis

If toxic erythema of the newborn becomes vesicular, it must be distinguished from staphylodermia. The latter, because of its infectiousness and possible complications (staphylococcal pneumonia, osteomyelitis, septicemia of the newborn) requires vigorous hygienic and therapeutic measures. These are not necessary in toxic erythema. Under the microscope, a methylene blue or Gram stain of the vesicular contents reveals staphylococci in pemphigoid and eosinophilic leukocytes in allergic bullosis.

Treatment

The exanthem will have disappeared spontaneously by the sixteenth day of life, so that treatment is unnecessary.

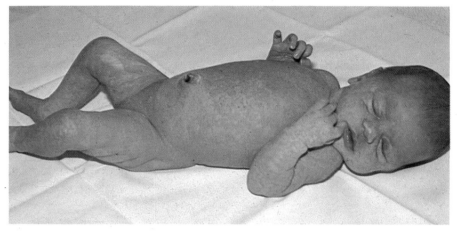

54 Four-day-old newborn showing slightly raised, morbilliform-confluent, toxic erythema.

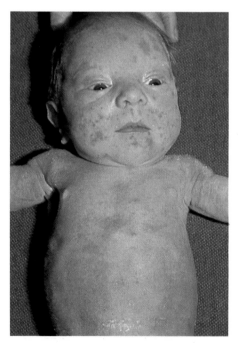

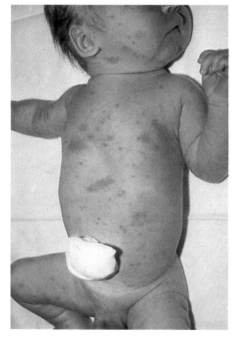

55 Erythema toxicum neonatorum on the tenth day of life.

56 Alternating urticarial-lichenoid-vesicular exanthem of the newborn from the first until the 14th day of life. Eosinophils in the blood are at 14 per cent.

Breast Engorgement of the Newborn

Definition

Breast engorgement of the newborn is caused by hypertrophy of the mammary glands. It begins with the third day of live, is found in 95 per cent of all infants and often accompanies secretion of colostrum. It may last from several weeks to months with a maximum during the second week of life. Maternal hormones are the causative agents (placental estrogens, prolactin of the anterior pituitary lobe), which have entered the fetal organism before labor (pregnancy reaction).

Clinical Findings

Only minor tenderness is present in hyperemic engorgement of the breast. In most cases the disorder is symmetrical, it increases in size until the middle of the second week of life, decreasing slowly thereafter. Pressure – which should be avoided – causes secretion of an opalescent fluid ("witch's-milk").

Differential Diagnosis

Both the female breast during lactation and the engorged breast of the newborn are susceptible to mastitis. Increased swelling with inflammatory rubor, locally elevated temperature, pain on pressure and finally fluctuation are warning signs (See p. 60).

Treatment

If need be, in the case of marked engorgement, a cottonwool dressing may be applied to prevent mechanical irritation. Regression occurs spontaneously within a few weeks, unless the glands are maltreated by squeezing out the colostrum, thus favoring infection and prolonging the duration of secretion. As in true lactation, emptying of the breast effects stimulation of lactation.

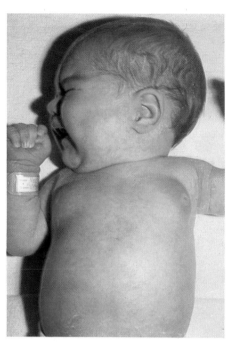

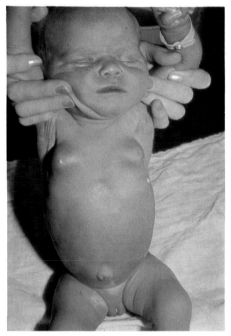

57 Ten-day-old female with bilateral mammary engorgement.

58 Pronounced hypertrophy of the mammary glands in an eight-day-old female. Note the discharge of "witch's milk" from the right nipple.

Umbilical Granuloma

Definition

Increased granulation tissue at the base of the umbilical wound (umbilical fungus) is called umbilical granuloma. Granulation impedes regular epithelization of the wound during the second to third week of life and causes persistent secretion (oozing umbilicus, umbilical blenorrhea).

Clinical Findings

The condition presents as a lentil to pea-sized, red, sessile or pedunculated granulation at the base of the umbilicus with a raspberrylike surface. Smaller granulomas often raise attention only by prolonged secretion and cannot be visualized before separation of the umbilical fold. Umbilical granuloma and oozing umbilicus are excellent ports of entry for infectious agents which may cause umbilical ulcer, omphalitis, peritonitis, sepsis, umbilical diphtheria and tetanus of the newborn.

Differential Diagnosis

Fistulas of the vitelline duct (persisting omphalomesenteric duct), Meckel's diverticulum communicating with the umbilicus and very infrequent urachal fistulas (persistent allantoic duct) may simulate umbilical granuloma. The diagnosis is verified by sounding the fistular orifice, testing the reaction of the secretion (intestinal fluid: alkaline, urine: generally acid), and filling the bladder with roentgen contrast medium or methylene blue solution.

Treatment

Umbilical granuloma is cauterized with silver nitrate and covered with a sterile dressing. Cauterization is painless because of the absence of nerve fibers in the granuloma. Pedunculated granulomas can be ligated with a silk thread.

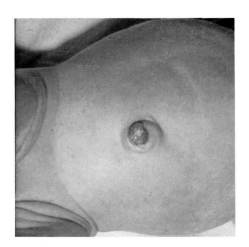

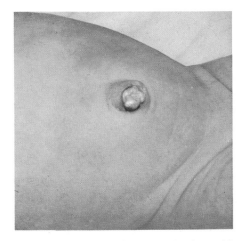

59 Umbilical granuloma with central powder remnants in a 14-day-old.

60 Immediately after cauterization with silver nitrate.

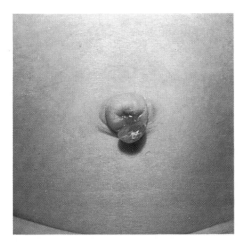

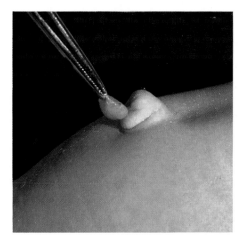

61 Pedunculated umbilical granuloma in a five-week-old.

62 Immediately before ligation.

Asphyxia

Definition

Asphyxia is the term for perinatal lack of oxygen in vital organs (hypoxia) accompanied by various complex functional disturbances of respiration (dyspnea, apnea) and circulation (stasis, cyanosis, diapedesis, bradycardia) of the central nervous system (areflexia) and of the acid-base balance (acidosis). The causes may be found either in the mother (prolonged pregnancy, erythroblastosis, lues, premature separation of the placenta, gestosis), during parturition (prolonged labor, placenta previa, breech presentation, forceps delivery, cesarean section, prolapse of the cord, anesthesia), or in the infant (cerebral, pulmonary, or cardiovascular asphyxia).

Clinical Findings

Intrauterine diagnosis of fetal asphyxia is based on the presence of fetal bradycardia below 100/min, by the loss of meconium verified by amnioscopy, by green amniotic fluid, and finally by acidosis proved by microblood examination. Postpartal symptomatology of *blue asphyxia* is characterized by apnea and cyanosis in spite of good cardiovascular (pulse, heart sounds) and neurologic (corneal reflex, muscle tone) conditions. With transition into *pale asphyxia* the color of the skin turns greycyanotic, circulation begins to fail, and muscle tone and reflexes disappear. The clinical signs can rapidly be assessed by the *Apgar score*. A score of zero to three indicates pale asphyxia, a score of four to six blue asphyxia.

Differential Diagnosis

Often clinical differentiation from cerebral hemorrhage, aspiration, atelectasis and posthemorrhagic shock is impossible. All these disorders may be causes or sequels of asphyxia.

Treatment

Clearing of the airways, oxygenation, keeping warm, and correction of acidosis are cardinal measures. Lethality is high and subsequent neurologic and mental defect syndromes are frequent.

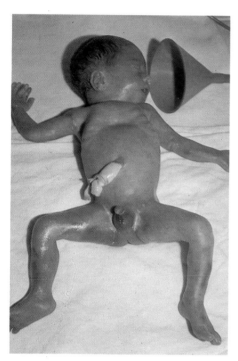

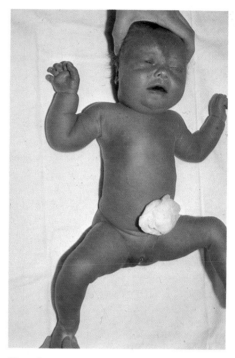

63   Premature infant (1450 g) immediately after delivery. The sternum retracts on inspiration owing to fetal atelectasis. Blue asphyxia predominates. Extensive cutaneous hemorrhage was caused by labor mechanics, immaturity, or hypoxia.

64   Post-term neonate with blue asphyxia. Apgar score: 5.

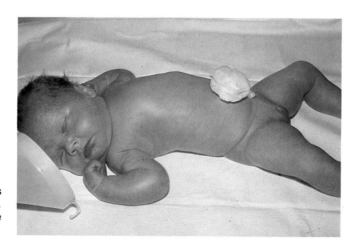

65   Subsiding cyanosis caused by oxygenation. Hypoxemic facial petechiae are evident.

Idiopathic Respiratory Distress Syndrome of the Newborn

Definition

The idiopathic respiratory distress syndrome of the newborn – or hyaline membrane syndrome – is a serious neonatal disturbance of respiration. Premature infants, infants after cesarean section, infants of diabetic mothers and second-born twins are mainly affected. Hypoxia and prematurity play the leading etiologic role. Pulmonary hyperemia, atelectasis, and hyaline membranes in the alveoli and bronchi, consisting of eosinophilic fibrin, are characteristic histologic findings. They are not, however, constant. Hyaline membrane disease is the main form of chronic postpartal asphyxia.

Clinical Findings

Clinical symptomatology starts a few hours after delivery with tachypnea over 65/min, inspiratory retraction (especially of the sternum), cyanosis and apneic attacks. Acidosis is the biochemical manifestation. On roentgenograms, there is a finely granulated cloudiness of the lung fields.

Differential Diagnosis

Respiratory disturbances caused by cerebral hemorrhage and hypoxia cannot always be differentiated from those of primary pulmonary origin such as hyaline membrane syndrome or aspiration.

Treatment

Symptomatic therapy must try to break through the vicious circle of hypoxia and membrane formation by means of massive oxygen supply and correction of acidosis. Still, one in two affected infants will die within the first three days of life.

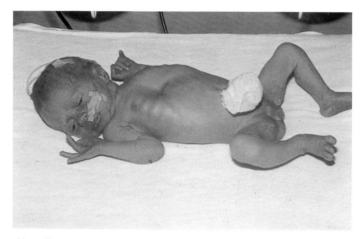

66   Three-day-old premature infant with respiratory distress syndrome. Birth weight 1970 g. At first, post-partal findings after cesarean section were normal. After six hours, severe apneic attacks and deep sternal retraction occurred. Here, in an oxygenated incubator, no cyanosis is present.

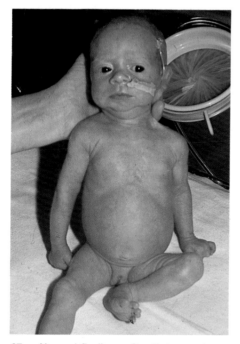

67   Normal findings after three weeks.

Melena Neonatorum

Definition

Hemorrhage from the gastrointestinal tract of the newborn, called true melena of the newborn, is the manifestation of neonatally disturbed adaptation of the blood clotting mechanism (hemorrhagic disease of the newborn). Hepatic prematurity, vitamin K deficiency caused by absent intestinal flora, insufficiency of prothrombin synthesis, thrombocytopenia, capillary fragility and hypoxia are among causative factors.

Clinical Findings

Bloodstained stools are discharged during the first week of life, most commonly during the second and fourth day. The color varies from black to bright red, depending on where the source of hemmorrhage is located in the intestinal tract and also depending on the age of the infant. In contrast to the blackish color of meconium, the stain of tarry stools in the diaper is surrounded by a red circle. Hematemesis may be present as well.

Differential Diagnosis

Melena spuria caused by swallowed blood in epistaxis or mamillary rhagades of the mother always appears as tarry stool. Symptomatic melena may be present in sepsis, syphilis and injuries of the anal mucosa, as for example those caused by a thermometer.

Treatment

Vitamin K supply is necessary and in serious cases blood transfusions may be required. But in most cases today the disease follows a mild course.

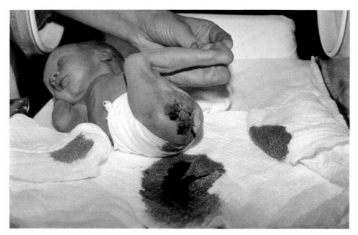

68   Melena neonatorum in a premature infant (1650 g) of five days. Healing was complete within three days owing to vitamin K administration (4 mg).

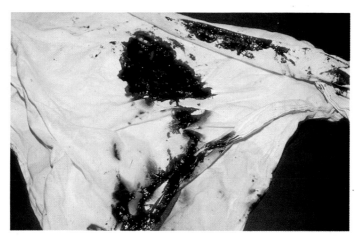

69   Melena with considerable hematemesis of a twin on the first day of life. After vitamin K administration, healing occurred by the fifth day of life.

Hemolytic Disease of the Newborn

Definition

The pathological principle of hemolytic disease of the newborn is hemolysis caused by reaction of maternal antibodies with blood factors of the infant, particularly Rh factor. This results in anemia, extramedullary hematopoiesis (erythroblastosis), hyperbilirubinemia and kernicterus. The morbidity of Rh erythroblastosis is about 0.5 per cent of all newborns. The frequency of ABO erythroblastosis is identical, but because of its often milder course, it comprises only about 20 per cent of the cases of clinically manifest hemolytic disease. Anti-D sensitization is the most frequent kind of Rh incompatibility; c, E and C sensitizations acount for four to five per cent.

Clinical Findings

1. In *hydrops fetalis,* hemolysis of fetal erythrocytes causes severe anemia with hypoxic myocardial and capillary damage, hypervolemia and generalized edema of fetus and placenta (hydrops universalis). Stillbirth will result in most of the cases.
2. In *icterus gravis,* the most common form of the disease, hemolysis leads to rapid postpartal rise of the bilirubin level and jaundice as early as the first or second day of life. During pregnancy, the fetal bilirubin is excreted by the mother. The newborn liver cannot adequately conju-

gate and eliminate bilirubin. If the critical bilirubin level of about 20 mg per 100 ml is exceeded, toxic damage to the basal ganglion will result (kernicterus, bilirubinencephalopathy).
3. In *anemia neonatorum,* anemia appearing in the second week of life is the only manifestation of hemolysis.

Differential Diagnosis

1. Physiologic jaundice of the newborn: appearing no earlier than the second day of life, generally on the third.
2. Jaundice of the premature infant.
3. Sepsis of the newborn.
4. Stress icterus caused by hemorrhage in traumatic birth.
5. Obstructive jaundice caused by atresia of bile ducts or the inspissated bile syndrome.
6. Hepatitis.
7. Familial hemolytic jaundice.

Treatment

The main purpose of treatment is to prevent kernicterus with its acute life-threatening and chronic encephalopathic sequels. This can be accomplished with near certainty if exchange transfusions are given in time. The diagrams of Polacek and Schellong are frequently used to establish indications (Figs. 70 and 71).

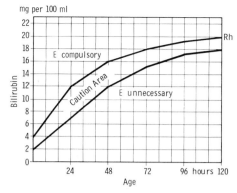

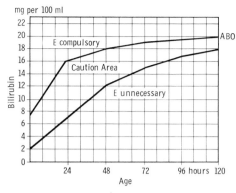

70 Diagram after Polacek demonstrating the indicators for exchange transfusion in hemolytic disease of the newborn caused by Rh incompatibility.

71 Modified diagram for use in hemolytic disease of the newborn caused by ABO incompatibility (Schellong 1968).

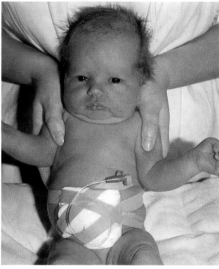

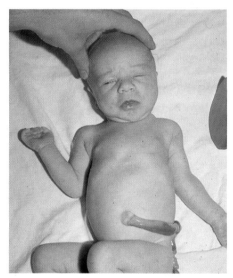

72 Rh erythroblastosis in a 24-hour-old neonate. Pink jaundice is evident, with serum bilirubin at 11 mg per 100 ml, anemia (erythrocytes at 3.9 million/μl), hemoglobin at 17.4 g per 100 ml, and reticulocytes at 11.1 per cent.

74 Severe Rh erythroblastosis of sixth infant immediately after delivery. Erythrocytes: 2.4 million/μl; Hb: 7.8 g per 100 ml; erythroblasts: 27; leukocytes: 34000/μL. Blood exchange provided the cure.

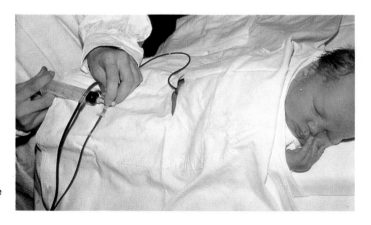

73 During exchange transfusion.

Sepsis of the Newborn

Definition

Sepsis of the newborn is a serious generalized bacterial infection. Premature and newborn infants are predisposed owing to immunologic insufficiency which is specific for early age. Staphylococci, meningococci, streptococci, pneumococci, hemophilus influenzae, Escherichia coli and pseudomonas aeruginosa (pyocyaneus) are among the causative organisms. Places of entry may be the umbilical wound, skin (pemphigoid), upper or lower respiratory tract (common rhinitis, aspiration), and intestinal mucosa.

Clinical Findings

Generally, clinical symptomatology starts in the second week of life and is often characteristic. Resistance to feeding, pallor, subicterus, vomiting, and diarrhea, are suggestive symptoms. Fever, enlargement of the spleen or leukocytosis may be absent. In fulminant cases, toxic hemorrhagic exanthems will appear. Different organic manifestations may result: purulent pneumonia, empyema, meningitis, osteomyelitis, phlegmon, cystitis with pyelonephritis, and peritonitis.

Differential Diagnosis

Septic cutaneous hemorrhage must not be mistaken for harmless toxic erythema of the newborn (See p. 44).

Treatment

Massive administration of antibiotics.

Prognosis

Primary infection is said to be responsible for two to fifteen per cent of neonatal mortality and may be a concomitant cause of death in 20 to 70 per cent. Today, with high doses of broad-spectrum antibiotics started early in the disease, lethality in neonatal sepsis is about 20 per cent.

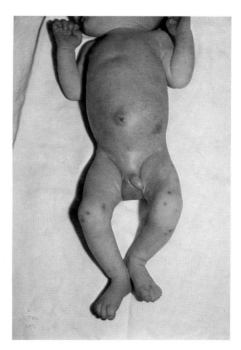

75   Umbilical sepsis in a 12-day-old newborn. Note the cyanotic color of the skin, toxic exanthem of the extremities, distended and tense abdomen, faint periumbilical reddening, and unremarkable external aspect of the umbilical wound. The condition was subfebrile, with leukocytes at 2400/µl and hematemesis; the outcome was fatal.

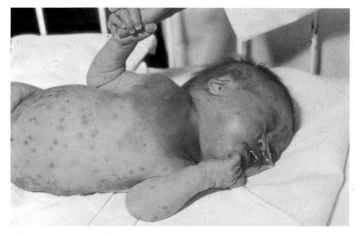

76   Left-sided phlegmon of the neck in a 14-day-old girl. Septic exanthem. Severe, afebrile illness with leukocytes at 4500/µl. Pus contained hemolytic staphylococci and staphylococcal pneumonia occurred. The outcome was fatal.

Mastitis Neonatorum

Definition

Mastitis in the newborn and in the young infant is a staphylococcal infection spreading in the milk ducts of the mammary gland. Frequently the disease is provoked by improper manipulation of harmless mammary engorgement of the newborn.

Clinical Findings

Local swelling, redness, elevated temperature and tenderness on palpation of one or both mammary glands precede suppuration.

Differential Diagnosis

Breast engorgement of the newborn as a reaction to pregnancy shows no inflammatory signs (See p. 46).

Treatment

If suppuration is not prevented in spite of antibiotic treatment, careful radial mamillary incision is indicated in order to avoid damage to lactiferous ducts.

Prognosis

In girls, suppurative mastitis neonatorum may later cause atrophy of the mammary glands.

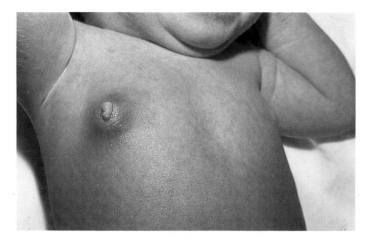

77   Suppurative right-sided mastitis in a 15-day-old girl. Spontaneous perforation and staphylococcus aureus were observed.

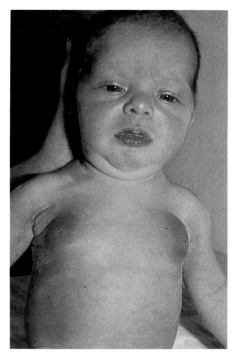

78   Bilateral mastitis neonatorum in a 12-day-old girl.

Phlegmon of the Scalp

Definition

In infants with lowered resistance phlegmon of the scalp may complicate sudoriparous abscesses of the occiput or may result from thrombophlebitis of cranial veins after continuous intravenous drip. Staphylococci and streptococci are the chief causative agents.

Clinical Findings

Expanded inflammatory edema of the scalp is present, changing its localization according to the position of the head. The edema originates from one or several sudoriparous abscesses in the scalp or from a thickened botuliform vein. Fluctuating pus expands beneath the scalp and is concomitant with diffuse heat swelling, and redness. Sepsis, osteomyelitis of the cranial bones and bacterial metastases to different organs are the most threatening complications.

Differential Diagnosis

Caput succedaneum, cephalhematoma (See p. 30), and osteomyelitis of cranial bones have to be excluded.

Treatment

Antibiotic therapy, supported by blood transfusions and nursing with human milk, is preferred. Pus is removed by large incision and contra-incision.

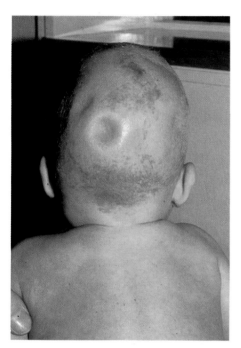 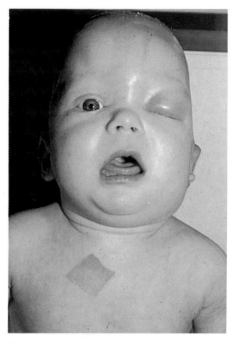

79 Beginning phlegmon of the scalp during the edematous stage, which occurred three days after a small sudoriparous abscess over the dorsal vertex area. Additional finding: nevus flammeus in the neck.

80 Concomitant edema of the upper eyelid after positioning the head to the left. Five days later, pus was evacuated through an occipital incision. Bacteriologic findings: staphylococcus aureus (haemolyticus).

Premature Twins

Definition

In general, the duration of twin pregnancy is shortened – by an average of 24 days. Even with normal duration, infants of multiple pregnancy usually are smaller and lighter than those of single pregnancy. Thus, with a birth weight of 2500 g or less, they are recorded as premature. The incidence of twin pregnancy is one in 80 to 90 pregnancies; 25 per cent of the twins are monozygotic, 75 per cent dizygotic. With growing maternal age the rate of twin pregnancies rises. Familial predisposition does exist.

Clinical Findings

Infants of multiple pregnancy show the characteristic anatomical and functional signs of prematurity: undersize, lanugo, absence of subcutaneous fat, and underdeveloped auricular cartilage, fingernails and genitalia. Central respiratory insufficiency, thermolability, absence of sucking and swallowing reflexes, extrapyramidal motoricity and hydrolability are also characteristic. Monozygotic twins are in danger of posthemorrhagic shock because of feto-fetal transfusion.

Treatment

Treatment is identical to the care of premature infants.

Prognosis

The second twin is more jeopardized by hypoxia than the first because of delayed delivery and frequent premature separation of the placenta. Additionally, in about one-third of the cases the infant is delivered by breech presentation. The lethality is twice as high as that of the first-born twin. Natal lethality of twins is reported as 10 to 20 per cent. Like permanent cerebral damage, it depends greatly on the degree of prematurity, i. e., the changes of survival are identical to those of premature infants:

About 600 g: possible viability;

  600 to 1000 g: mortality about 90 per cent;

1000 to 1500 g: mortality about 50 per cent;

1500 to 2000 g: mortality about 25 per cent;

2000 to 2500 g: mortality about 10 per cent.

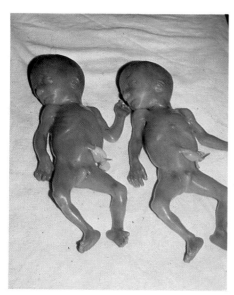

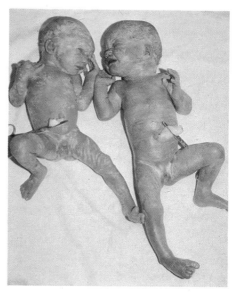

81   Premature twins, 490 and 500 g after a 22-week-gestation. Shiny, transparent skin, and all signs of immaturity are present. Death occurred from central respiratory failure after two hours.

82   Premature twins, 1550 and 2150 g. Slight cyanosis occurred in the second-born. Vernix caseosa.

Nutritional Disturbances

Dyspepsia

Definition

The less severe form of acute diarrhea in the newborn is called dyspepsia. Pathogenetically this is acute digestive insufficiency. It may be caused by parenteral infections by viruses or bacteria, from infections of the upper respiratory tract, otitis, and pneumonia; intestinal infections by coli bacteria, staphylococci, pseudomonas aeruginose (pyocyaneus), salmonellae (typhoid and paratyphoid, see typhimurium), shigellae (Sonne); or by feeding faults, e. g., dyspepsia of ablactation and change of nutrition. Beyond infancy, acute diarrhea is called enteritis or gastroenteritis.

Clinical Findings

Diarrhea is the cardinal symptom of dyspepsia: increased number of liquid stools up to spurting evacuation. Prodromic signs are restlessness, lack of appetite, and gluteal intertrigo. Weight loss, vomiting, and decreased turgor of the skin complete the picture of dyspepsia. The slow return of lifted abdominal skin reveals decreased cutaneous turgor.

Treatment

Treatment consists of dietetic measures and antibiotic therapy.

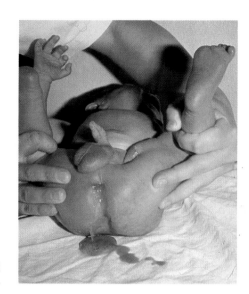

83 Spurting liquid stools in a 20-day-old infant with a periproctitic abscess and dyspepsia.

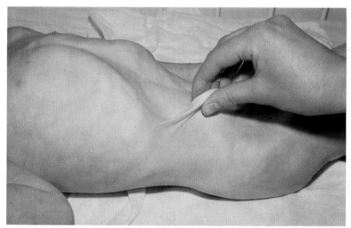

84 Decreased turgor of the skin in parenteral dyspepsia.

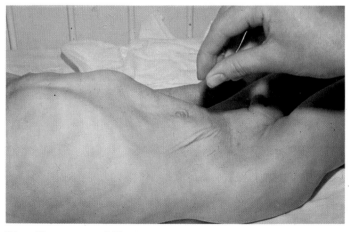

85 Slow return of lifted abdominal skin.

Subtoxic Dyspepsia

Definition

As fluid loss (dehydration) increases, dyspepsia turns into a serious clinical disorder characterized by major signs of exsiccosis (sub or pretoxic dyspepsia).

Clinical Findings

Besides diarrhea and vomiting, the following signs of dehydration are prominent: loss of turgor, retracted fontanels, sunken eyes, dry lips and tongue, and retracted abdomen. The skin is pale and cool, respiration deepened and, after initial excitement, apathy sets in.

Treatment

Dietetic and antibiotic treatment complemented by parenteral application of fluids and correction of acidosis by intravenous drip.

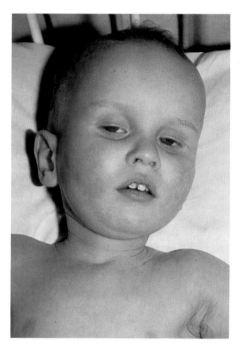

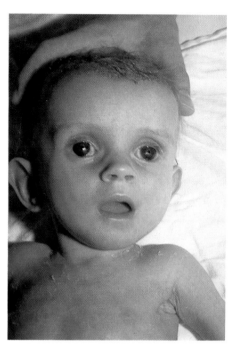

86 Subtoxic dyspepsia in catarrhal otitis media. The 13-month-old boy is apathetic and near collapse. The lips are dry, with withered axillary skin.

87 Pretoxic dyspepsia in a five-month-old infant. Lethargy, dehydration, acidosis and circulatory failure presided. Pallor occurred despite a fever of 39°C.

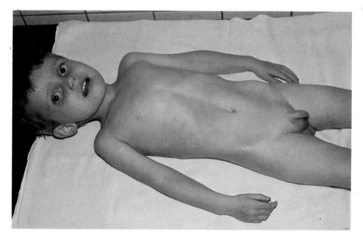

88 Pretoxic diarrhea and vomiting in a 30-month-old boy. Note the frightened facial expression, greyish-pale color of the skin, sunken bulbi, dry lips, slowed respiration, and retracted abdomen. Alternating restlessness and somnolence.

Intoxication

Definition

Intoxication (toxicosis, dyspeptic coma) is the most serious form of acute diarrhea of the newborn. The sequence of dehydration, hypovolemia, and hypoxia, as well as viral-bacterial and endogenous formation of toxins, lead to life-threatening disturbances of vital functions in intermediary metabolism, circulation and the central nervous system.

Clinical Findings

Beside considerable weight loss, disturbance of consciousness from somnolence to stupor to coma, and acidotic breathing (Kussmaul's respiration) are the major signs. Dehydration of varying intensity may be present: doughy skin, retracted fontanels, sunken eyes, scaphoid abdomen, and hypovolemic circulatory shock. Central nervous signs include initial irritation with "cri encéphalique"; later, lack of motion, rare blinking, congested sclerae, a vacant expression and limited consciousness. Acetonemia, acidosis, and hypokalemia are the biochemical changes causing the relevant clinical conditions.

Differential Diagnosis

Fulminant development of the central nervous signs of intoxication with hyperpyrexia (disregarding the dyspeptic and pretoxic stage) and encephalitis caused by enteroneurotropic viruses. The prognosis is poor.

Treatment

The principles of the treatment of toxicosis consist of prompt intravenous substitution of fluids and electrolytes, control of acidosis and administration of antibiotics and cortisone.

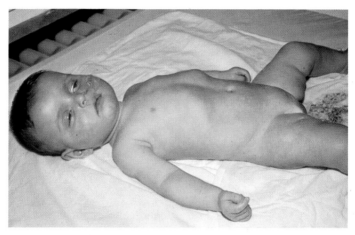

89   Intoxication in a five-month-old with pertussis. Watery stools in diaper, scaphoid abdomen, livid pallor, unconsciousness, mask face, and traces of cold sweat indicating circulatory insufficiency occurred.

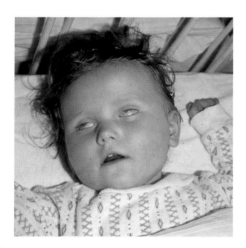

90   Dyspeptic coma in a twelve-month-old girl. Pallor, dry lips, and injected conjunctiva are evident. Illness began two days previously with fever, vomiting and diarrhea.

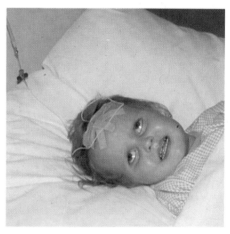

91   Toxic gastroenteritis in a 23-month-old girl. Note the vacant, unconscious expression in the large, sunken eyes. The infant fell ill with diarrhea and vomiting two days previously.

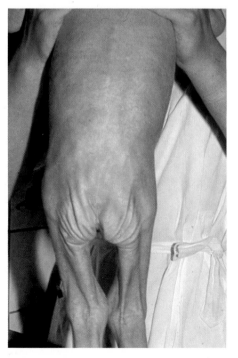

Dystrophy and Atrophy

Definition

Dystrophy is the less severe and atrophy the serious form of chronic growth retardation caused by malnutrition. It may be caused by insufficient exogenous food supply, deficient digestion (mucoviscidosis, disaccharide malabsorption) or disturbed absorption of nutritional substances (celiac disease, glucose-galactose malabsorption). Serious organic damage to heart, brain, or kidney may also cause cardial, cerebral, or renal dystrophy. Today, chronic recurrent infections like occult mastoiditis rarely cause dystrophy.

92 Dyscerebral atrophy in a 22-month-old infant: marked weight loss, relatively large head, broad mouth, weight 6000 g.

Clinical Findings

Relative loss of weight owing to deficient weight gain is the cardinal sign of *dystrophy*. Shrinking of subcutaneous fat tissue creates the picture of the large abdomen with flaccid abdominal walls and tobacco-pouch buttocks. In addition, there is a predisposition to acute dyspepsia, and resistance against infections is lowered. The clinical picture of *atrophy* is characterized by skeleton-like emaciation with senile features and depression of all vital functions. In the final state of complete decomposition, life fades away under the signs of central respiratory and circulatory failure.

Treatment

Dietetic treatment is directed according to the respective causes of dystrophy or atrophy.

93 Tobacco-pouch buttocks.

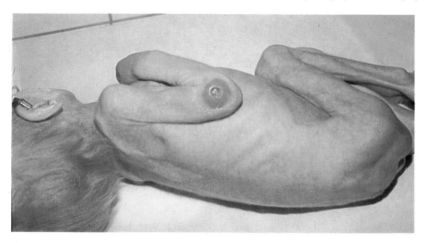

94   The torpid reel-ringed ecthyma of the atrophic child is deeply punched out, and appears mainly on sites exposed to pressure.

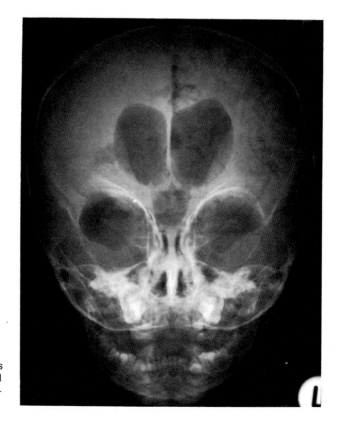

95   Hydrocephalus internus et externus e vacuo in cerebral atrophy is a causative or concomitant factor of atrophy.

Disturbances of Growth, Metabolism, the Endocrine System

Primordial Dwarfism

Definition

Primordial dwarfism is the manifestation of direct, genetically determined false regulation of skeletal growth. Occurrence is sporadic or familial and no other dysplasias or endocrine deficiencies are present. As in all forms of growth retardation, a reduction of body length between two and three sigma compared to the average, is called microsomia; a reduction of more than three sigma, dwarfism (nasosomia). Reduction up to two sigma (double standard deviation) compared to the average is within range of normal variation.

Clinical Findings

A congenital, well-proportioned, small size of the individuum is the striking symptom of primordial dwarfism. Even at birth the infants are undersized in spite of full term pregnancy. Skeletal age, mental development, and onset of puberty correspond to actual age.

Differential Diagnosis

Descriptive differentiation from hypopituitary growth retardation may be difficult, since the latter also goes along with well-proportioned size and undisturbed development of intelligence. At birth, however, hypopituitary dwarfs are of normal size and weight. Growth retardation becomes manifest in the third year of life and skeletal age is retarded (See p. 78).

Treatment

There are no therapeutic possibilities.

Prognosis

The children do not reach the size of normal adults. Further development and life expectancy are normal.

Somatogram

Year		cm	±2σ	kg	±2σ
5	—	114	±9	19,6	±4,0
	—	113		19,2	
	—	112		18,8	
	—	111		18,4	
	—	110		18,0	
		109		17,6	
4	—	108	±8	17,3	±3,5
	—	107		17,0	
	—	106		16,7	
	—	105		16,4	
	—	104		16,1	
		103		15,8	
3	—	102	±7	15,5	±2,9
	—	101		15,3	
	—	100		15,1	
	—	99		14,9	
	—	98		14,7	
	—	97		14,5	
	—	96		14,3	
		95		14,1	
2½	—	94	±7	13,9	±2,9
	—	93		13,7	
	—	92		13,5	
		91		13,3	
2	—	90	±7	13,1	±2,7
	—	89		12,9	
	—	88		12,7	
	—	87		12,5	
		86		12,3	
1½	—	85	±7	12,1	±2,5
	—	84		11,9	
	—	83		11,7	
	—	82		11,5	
	—	81		11,3	
	—	80		11,1	
1	—	79	±6	10,9	±2,3
	—	78		10,7	
	—	77		10,5	
	—	76		10,3	
	—	75		10,1	
		74		9,8	
	11	73	±5	9,5	±1,8
	10	72		9,2	
	9	71		8,8	
	8	70		8,4	
½	7	68		8,0	
	6	66		7,5	
	5	64	±4	7,0	±1,5
	4	62		6,4	±1,5
	3	59		5,6	±1,2
	2	56		4,8	±1,2
	1	53		3,9	±0,9
	0	50		3,3	±0,8

Girl   **97**

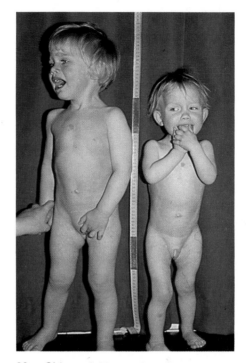

96   Girl aged 23 months, with primordial growth retardation compared to a normal child of the same age. The body structure is well proportioned; psyche corresponding to age.

97   Somatogram of the infant: birth weight 2700 g; birth length two weeks over term: 49 cm. Mother (155 cm) and maternal grandfather were both small.

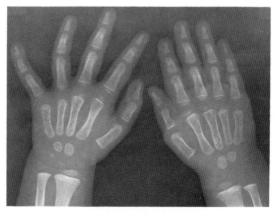

98   A typical radiogram of primordial growth retardation, as demonstrated in the above infant. Chronologic age 23 months, bone age two years, age according to length of hand (length of hand 100 mm) 15 months.

Diabetic Coma

Definition

Diabetic coma is a hyperglycemic-keto-acidotic decompensation of metabolism in diabetes mellitus, accompanied by disturbed consciousness. It is caused by faulty diet, deficient insulin administration, or acute infections.

Clinical Findings

Diabetic coma develops from a pre-comatose state with fatigue, lack of appetite, thirst, upper abdominal complaints, and vomiting. Consciousness is increasingly clouded until the full picture of diabetic coma is established, showing areflexia, acidotic respiration (Kussmaul), acetone odor, dehydration (soft bulbi, dry skin and mucous membranes), and circulatory failure. Diagnosis is confirmed by proof of hyperglycemia (400 to 1000 mg per 100 ml), glycosuria, and ketonuria.

Differential Diagnosis

Nausea, vomiting, and abdominal complaints may lead to the faulty diagnosis of an acute intra-abdominal process. Surgery would be disastrous. Meningitis or encephalitis, acetonemic vomiting and hypoglycemic shock have to be excluded (Table 1).

Table 1. Differential Diagnosis of Hyper and Hypoglycemia.

Diabetic Coma	Hypoglycemic Shock
Slow development	Sudden appearance
Kussmaul's respiration	Normal respiration
Dry skin	Moist skin
Soft bulbi	Firm bulbi
Soft, rapid pulse	Normal pulse
Hyporeflexia	Hyperreflexia to convulsions

Treatment

Immediate hospitalization is imperative. Continuous intravenous infusion of short-acting insulin, fluids, electrolytes (Na, K, Cl), and glucose.

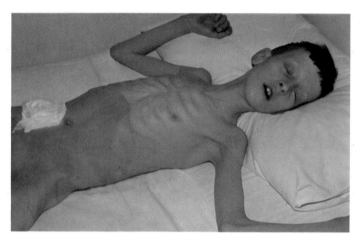

99   Boy in diabetic coma, age 9³/₄ years. Weight loss, scaphoid abdomen, Kussmaul's respiration, dry skin and lips, and slight cyanosis owing to circulatory insufficiency were noted. Excessive thirst and polyuria occurred for six weeks; appendectomy was performed on the previous day because of abdominal complaints and vomiting.

Hypopituitarism

Definition

Pituitary dwarfism is caused by lack of somatotropic hormone owing to insufficiency of the anterior lobe of the pituitary gland. Pathogenetically, recessive hereditary transmission, cerebral birth trauma, or tumors (craniopharyngioma) may be responsible. In the majority of cases, the etiology remains unclear.

Clinical Findings

Well-proportioned growth retardation along with normal development of intelligence becomes evident in most cases after the second year of age. Acromicria, doll-face, and slight obesity of the trunk are distinctive signs. Roentgenograms of the hand show characteristic equal retardation of ossification centers and longitudinal growth (Table 2). The diagnosis is confirmed by the insulin tolerance test, nitrogen retention test, metopirone test, and direct determination of somatotropic hormone in the plasma.

Differential Diagnosis

Table 2 shows some conditions to be included in the differential diagnosis. Constitutional growth retardation and primordial growth retardation are more common than deficiency of somatotropic hormone.

Treatment

Long-term parenteral administration of human growth hormone.

Prognosis

Without hormonal substitution, a final body length of 130 to 140 cm will be reached. Absence of sexual maturity proves simultaneous absence of gonadotropin production.

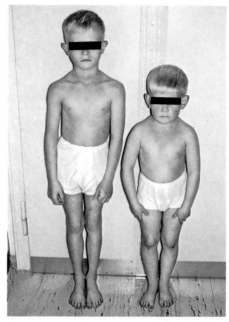

100 Eight-year-old boy with pituitary dwarfism compared to normal child of the same age. Body length 105 cm, weight 19.5 kg. Infantile proportions, round contours.

Table 2. Longitudinal Age and Bone Age in Several Types of Growth Retardation

	Longitudinal age	Bone age
Primordial dwarfism	delayed	corresponding to age
Pituitary dwarfism	delayed	delayed
Dwarfism in hypothyroidism	delayed	considerably delayed
Pubertas praecox	increased	advanced
Pseudopubertas praecox	increased	considerably advanced

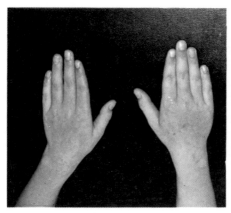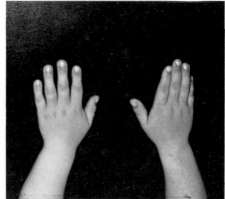

101   Acromicria of the infant (compared with hands corresponding to age).

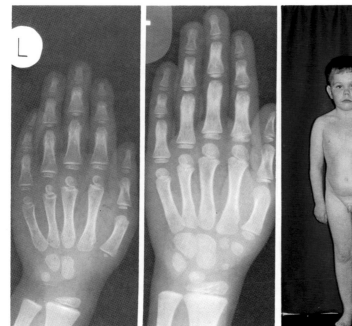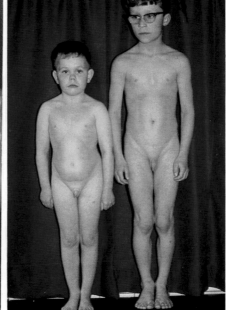

102   Osseous age of the child with pituitary dwarfism shown in Figs. 100 and 101 at three and one-half years, compared with radiogram of normal child at the same age.

103   Pituitary dwarfism in a boy aged 9 years, ten months. Body length: 106 cm; doll-face; osseous age, five and one-half years.

Hypothyroidism

Definition

Most of the cases of congenital hypothyroidism are caused by genetically unknown aplasia (athyroidism) or hypoplasia (hypothyroidism) of the thyroid gland. In addition, there are cases of hypothyroidism originating in defective iodine metabolism owing to congenital enzymatic disturbances and secondary hypothyroidism accompanying hypophyseal growth retardation (lack of thyrotrophic hormone). In children, acquired hypothyroidism is rare.

Clinical Findings

Generally, congenital hypothyroidism will not become evident until a few weeks after delivery. It may be preceded by prolonged jaundice. Lazy feeding, lack of motion, somnolence, and constipation are striking functional signs. Macroglossia, scanty course hair, and dry myxedematous skin are distinctive manifestations. The dwarfism is disproportionate, dental and osseous formation and physical and mental development are retarded. The diagnosis is confirmed by roentgenograms of the hand, electrocardiogram (low voltage), low serum level of protein-bound iodine (PBI) and tri-iodothyronine (T_3 test), reduced alkaline phosphatase, and, beyond infancy hypercholesteremia.

Differential Diagnosis

Down's syndrome, pituitary dwarfism, chondrodystrophy, and dysostosis multiplex (Pfaundler-Hurler) have to be excluded.

Treatment

Lifelong oral administration of thyroid hormone is necessary.

Prognosis

Prognosis depends on the degree of functional disturbance and commencement of treatment. Chances of somatic development are better than those of intellectual growth. One-third to one-half of the children treated for congenital hypo or athyroidism are oligophrenic. Acquired and secondary hypothyroidism do not affect intelligence.

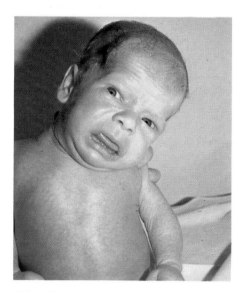

104 Two-month-old infant with hypothyroidism: coarse features, sparse hair, retracted root of nose, large tongue, pale yellow skin, sleepiness, poor drinking, decreased motion, hypothermia, hoarse crying.

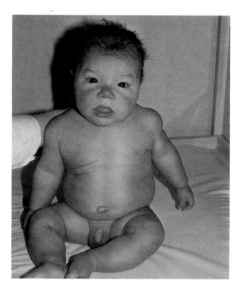

105 Hypothyroidism in a ten-month-old infant. Evident are typical myxedematous aspect, doughy swelling of subcutaneous tissue, shaggy hair, enlarged tongue, apathy, constipation, and hypothermia.

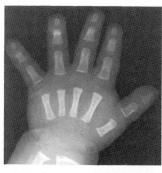
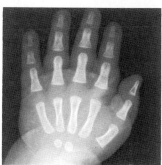

106 Radiologically empty carpal space of ten-month-old infant compared with normal hand of a healthy infant of the same age.

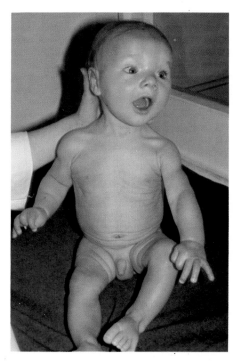

107 Six weeks after commencing treatment with thyroid extract, the aspect and behavior of the infant shown in Fig. 105 have changed completely and appear normal.

Goiter

Definition

In most cases, infantile goiter is a diffuse, parenchymatous hyperplasia of the thyroid gland without hormonal disturbances (atoxic, euthyroid goiter). Incidence is highest in newborns, infants, and in puberty. Different factors may lead to latent deficiency in thyroid hormone: lack of iodine, hereditary disturbance of hormonal synthesis, disordered iodine metabolism. In goiter of the newborn, disease of the maternal thyroid may be a causative factor. Thus, the pituitary feedback mechanism causes increased stimulation and hyperplasia of the thyroid gland.

Clinical Findings

Swallowing causes the soft and enlarged thyroid gland to move up and down. During school age, cystic-nodular changes may be present. In the newborn, respiration may be impeded, manifested by cyanosis, congenital stridor, difficulties in swallowing, and vomiting. Different from thymic stridor, stridor caused by goiter occurs predominantly in inspiration and decreases with reclination of the head.

Treatment

Goiter caused by lack of iodine is treated with potassium iodide, and disturbances of hormonal synthesis with thyroid hormone. The prognosis is favorable. During childhood, thyroidectomy is seldom indicated.

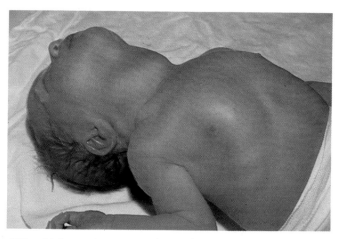

108   Male newborn with congenital struma. Complete regression within six weeks under treatment with 5 per cent potassium iodide ointment. The mother had been affected with euthyroid struma since the age of twelve, showing a recrudescence with every new pregnancy.

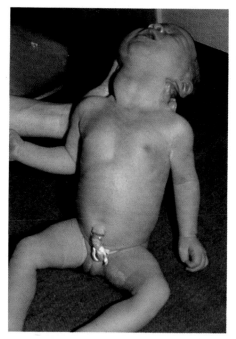

109   Newborn girl with large congenital struma. Palpation indicates diffuse, soft swelling of the right lobe of the thyroid gland; somewhat less pronounced on the left side. Good response to percutaneous administration of iodide, with regression occurring within four weeks.

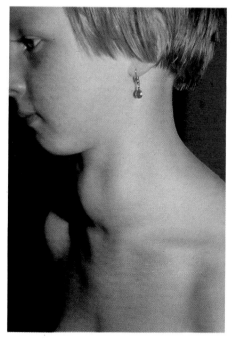

110   Hyperthyroid girl, aged nine years, seven months, with euthyroid, prepuberal struma.

Turner's Syndrome

Definition

Turner's syndrome is the term for a complex of malformations always characterized by gonadal dysgenesis. In most cases the underlying cause is a chromosomal aberration, typified by the absence of one sex chromosome (monosomic, XO disorder). XO constellation is present in one percent of fertilized oocytes, but abortion occurs in a very high percentage. Thus, the incidence of Turner's syndrome in newborn girls is 1:3000.

Clinical Findings

The phenotype is female, gonads are absent, and edema of the dorsum of hands and feet may be present at birth. With growing age there are: growth retardation, broad chest (scutiform thorax) with increased intermamillary distance, webbed neck, low nuchal hair line, masculine features, cubitus valgus, and often pigmented nevi. Later, development of the breast is absent and menstruation will not appear (primary amenorrhea). Diagnosis: sex, chromatin-negative (male) which is found in 80 per cent of the cases, and chromosomal analysis, karyotype 45, X.

Treatment

Administration of estrogens; psychological guidance beyond the first decade of life constitutes the most difficult therapeutic problem.

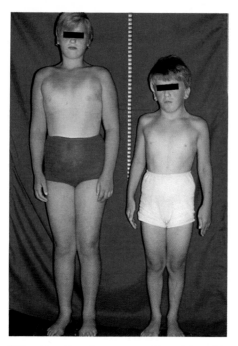

111 Small eleven-year-old girl with Turner's syndrome compared to normal child of the same age: body length 128 cm, hypoplastic nipples, scutiform chest, pyknic stature.

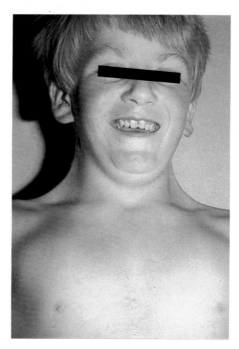

112 Pterygium colli, coarse features.

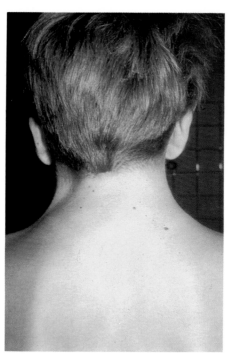

113 Short neck, low nuchal hairline.

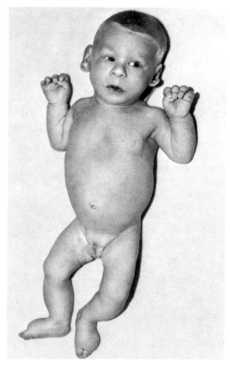

114 Four-week-old child with Turner's syndrome (Karyotype 45, XO).

Infectious Diseases

BCG-Vaccination

Definition

Vaccination for tuberculosis is an active immunization by a bovine tubercle strain which after repeated culture has become attenuated (Bacille Calmette-Guérin). Immunologically this corresponds to primary natural infection as shown by positive tuberculin tests six to eight weeks later. Just as natural infection, vaccination will only cause relative immunity.

Clinical Findings

After intracutaneous injection (left thigh) the intradermal weal disappears within a few minutes. After two to three weeks a bluish-red, pea-sized nodule will develop, which may liquefy or ulcerate. A lasting scar has been formed after four months. Swelling of regional lymph nodes may occur, liquefaction of inguinal lymph nodes is rare.

Complications

If ulceration occurs at the site of vaccination, bathing of the infant is stopped in order to avoid unspecific superinfection, which also might cause inguinal lymphadenitis. The site of vaccination is covered with dry sterile dressings.

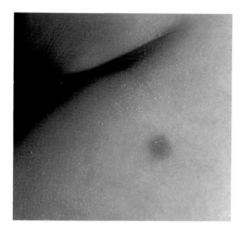

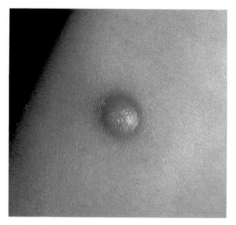

115   Normal BCG-vaccination nodule eight weeks after vaccination.

116   Pea-sized liquefaction at the site of vaccination three months later.

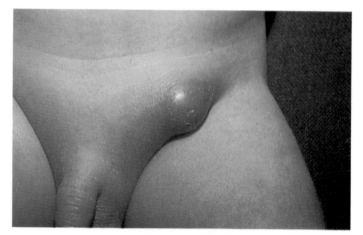

117   Suppurative inguinal lymphadenitis nine weeks after BCG vaccination. Probably unspecific superinfection at the site of BCG vaccination. The lymph nodes contained staphylococcal pus. After spontaneous perforation, uncomplicated healing occurred within two weeks.

Vaccination against Smallpox

Definition

Variolization – inaugurated by Edward Jenner in 1798 – is an active immunization with a smallpox virus which has been attenuated by passage through many generations of animals. It is performed as primary vaccination during the first three years of life and is repeated with booster effect in the twelfth year of life at the latest.

Clinical Findings

Three days after primary vaccination, a papule develops at the site of vaccination followed by an umbilicated pustule which is surrounded by an areola. Finally, on further drying, a crust forms which is shed after three weeks leaving a scar. Between the eighth and twelfth day a febrile reaction occurs. In revaccination, the extent of reaction (nodule, vesicle, or small pustule) corresponds to the grade of immunity present.

Complications

1. Unspecific infections because of transitory lowered vaccination-induced resistance.
2. Local gangrenous vaccinia (e.g., in secondary infection or antibody deficiency syndrome).
3. Secondary vaccinia caused by scratching the primary lesion and transfer to defective epithelium at a different site of the body.
4. Inoculation or translocation vaccinia caused similarly in another nonimmune person.
5. Generalized vaccinia by hematogenic dissemination.
6. Eczema vaccinatum in eczematous children caused by hematogenic dissemination.
7. Postvaccinal encephalitis with a morbidity of one to two in 20,000 infants having undergone primary vaccination. The complication appears during the first three years of life, with a mortality of 25 to 30 per cent.

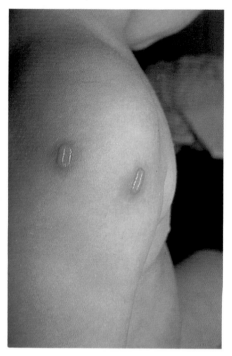

118   Normal umbilical pustule seven days after primary smallpox vaccination.

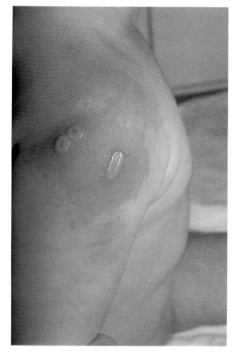

119   Three vaccination pustules with marked areola seven days after primary vaccination.

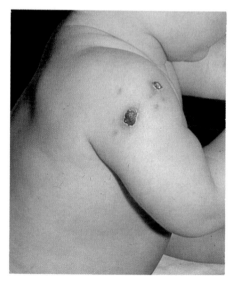

120   Vaccination crusts shortly before shedding four weeks after primary vaccination.

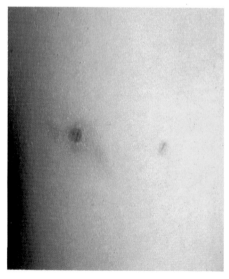

121   Normal nodular reaction of a twelve-year-old child seven days after revaccination.

Palpebral Vaccinia

Definition

If calf lymph is transmitted from the site of vaccination to the eye, pustules may develop on the eyelid (palpebral vaccinia), on the conjunctiva (conjunctival vaccinia) or on the cornea (corneal vaccinia).

Clinical Findings

Vaccinia of the eye also causes palpebral pustules, edema, chemosis, discharge, itching, and blepharospasm.

Treatment

Palpebral vaccinia heals simultaneously with the pustules at the site of vaccination. Healing is promoted by administration of gamma-globulin, vaccinal hyperimmune serum and antibiotics in order to prevent superinfection.

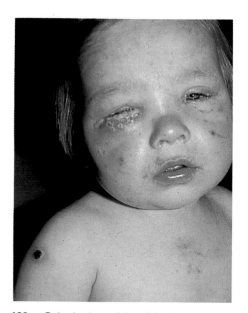

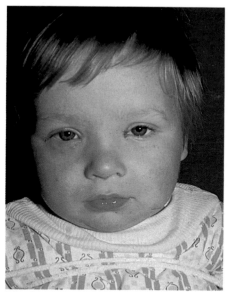

122 Palpebral vaccinia of the right side 18 days after primary smallpox vaccination: multiple pustules, palpebral edema, secretion, vaccination crust on the right humerus. Papulous postvaccinal exanthem over the sternum.

123   Improvement one week later.

Measles (MORBILLI — RED MEASLES)
↳ RUBEOLA

Definition

ID 10-14

Morbilli is a highly communicable disease caused by myxoviruses. The infectious agents enter the organism via conjunctivae and the upper respiratory tract. The incubation period is ten days. The disease follows a fixed scheme of prodromal and exanthematous manifestations and causes lifelong immunity.

Clinical Findings

The febrile-catarrhal prodromal stage consists of conjunctivitis, rhinitis, bronchitis, enanthem, and Koplik's spots. The exanthematous stage follows after three days with repeated rise of temperature: small blotchy skin eruptions eventually increase in size. They first appear on the cranial portions of the body and spread caudally. They coalesce into larger hemorrhagic patches and fade within a week following the same sequence as on initial appearance. Infectiousness is highest during the prodromal stage and ceases more or less after the third day of the exanthem.

Treatment

Treatment is symptomatic. The course may be mitigated by administration of gamma-globulin during the prodromal stage.
↳ passive immuni.

Prophylaxis

Vaccination gains increasing importance because of possible complications such as bronchopneumonia, croup-like manifestations and, most of all, encephalitis (frequency 1:1000, fatal course in 10 to 20 per cent, permanent sequelae in 30 per cent. The live-virus vaccine may be administered after the ninth month of life.

incubation : 10d

CATARRHAL STAGE. (HIGHLY INFECTIOUS)
- acute febrile onset
  - nasal catarrh
  - sneezing
  - redness of conjunctiva
  - swelling of eyelids
  - watery eyes
  - cough
on 2nd day: [- hoarseness 2° to laryngitis
             [- photophobia

- see KOPLIK SPOTS
- child irritable + miserable

EXANTHEMATOUS STAGE
- 3-4d after catarrhal stage Koplik spots disappear
- macular or maculopapular develops:
  - starts on back of ear + at junction of the forehead + the hair
  - in a few hrs there invasion of the wh skin
  - spots rapidly become more numerous + fo to form blotchy appearance.

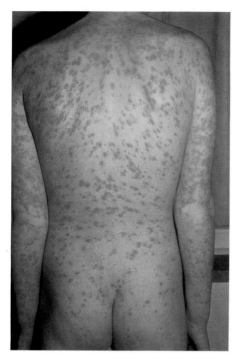

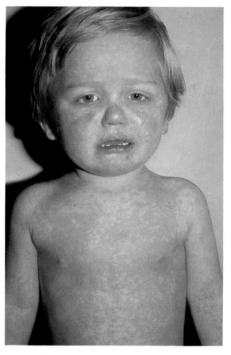

124 Typical marked measles rash with large macules. Second exanthematous day.

125 Confluent measles eruptions on the second exanthematous day.

- face most densely covered area.
- rash fully erupted in 2-3 d
+ then begins to fade
into a faint brown staining
+ fine desquamation of the
skin

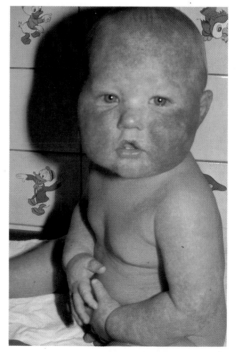

126 Hemorrhagic measles exanthem.

German Measles

Definition

Rubella is a viral, exanthematous, infectious disease with an incubation period of two to three weeks. The clinical course — simulating rudimentary measles — is mild and in many cases unapparent or unrecognized. The disease causes lifelong immunity. During the first two decades of life the incidence exceeds 80 per cent. There is one fact of major importance: if rubella occurs in pregnant women during the first trimester, abortion (10 to 15 per cent of cases) or fetal anomalies (22 to 35 per cent, embryopathy of rubella) may result.

Clinical Findings

After a discrete, catarrhal prodrome, the first manifestation is appearance of a rash in the face. The morphological appearance of the exanthem lies between that of measles and scarlet fever: fine, pale-red, isolated macules which disappear after one to three days. Occipital and cervical lymphadenopathy, leukopenia with relative lymphocytosis, and an increased number of plasma cells are typical findings.

Differential Diagnosis

Measles, scarlet fever, echovirus exanthem, exanthem subitum, infectious mononucleosis and allergic exanthematous reactions have to be excluded.

Treatment

Treatment is not required.

Prophylaxis

In order to prevent embryopathy, it is advisable to expose girls to natural infection before sexual maturity or to have them vaccinated with live attenuated rubella vaccine.

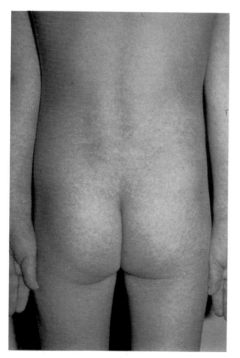

127   Rubella exanthem. First exanthematous day.

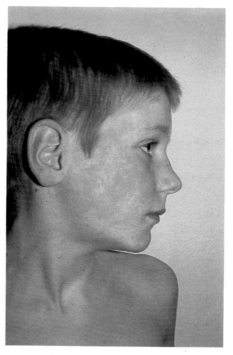

128   Fully developed rubella exanthem in the face on the second exanthematous day.

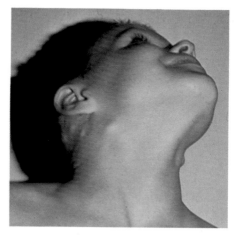

129   Swelling of the occipital, retroauricular, and submandibular lymph nodes in rubella on the third day of illness. Exanthem already faded.

Chickenpox (VARICELLA) — herpesvirus —

Definition

Chickenpox or varicella is a highly infectious, exanthematous disease of childhood. It is caused by the same virus as zoster, appears without prodrome after an incubation period of two to three weeks and causes lifelong immunity.

Clinical Findings

Accompanied by slightly raised temperature, red spots develop into nodes and pustules as large as a pea. The duration of the process is not always the same. Occasionally a scanty erythema may be noticed (varicella rash). The lesions tend to appear in crops. As early as a few hours later, the typical, polymorphous state of so-called "Heubner's celestial map" may be present, showing all stages and sizes of lesions at the same time and in the same vicinity. Contrary to strophulus, the exanthem of varicella also spreads over scalp and mucous membranes, and contrary to smallpox, palms and soles are not affected. Occasionally the pustules are umbilicated; they will dry up, form crusts and cause considerable itching. Scratching readily causes superinfection. Infectiousness is believed to be present until the scabs have fallen off.

Differential Diagnosis

Strophulus efflorescences (nodules and pustules) are not found on the scalp or mucous membranes. In smallpox, there is a prodrome of two to four days with high temperature and severe malaise. Then, with falling and again rising temperature, the smallpox exanthem will appear. This shows a monomorphous appearance during every single phase: spots followed by papules, vesicles after the third exanthematous day, pustules after the fourth day, umbilicated pustules after the seventh and crusts after the ninth day.

Treatment

Antipruritic powder, and prevention of scratching and subsequent superinfection are favored techniques.

- INCUBATION PERIOD 14-21d
- rash - appears on trunk → 2nd d of illness
   - then the face.
   - finally the limbs

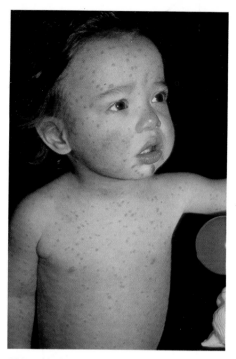

130 Varicella on second day of rash. Predominantly macules and papules, but also beginning vesiculation.

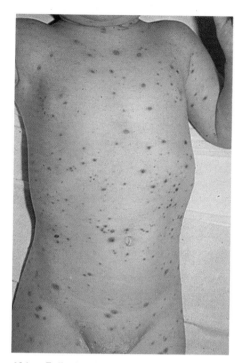

131 Fully developed typical polymorphous eruptive manifestations of varicella on the fifth exanthematous day.

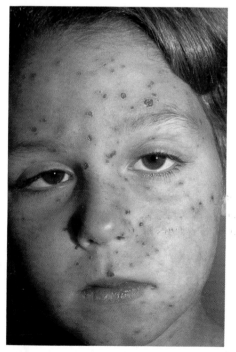

132 On the sixth exanthematous day most of the efflorescences have dried and crusts have been formed.

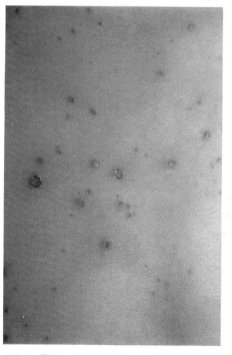

133 Heubner's "celestial map" on the sixth exanthematous day: macules, nodules, vesicles, umbilicated vesicles, pustules, and crusts lie side by side.

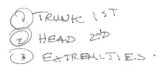

① TRUNK 1ST
② HEAD 2ND
③ EXTREMITIES.

Thoracic Phlegmon in Chickenpox

Definition

Gangrenous, necrotizing, or phlegmonous varicella may follow bacterial infection owing to scratching of varicella vesicles. Previously damaged skin (eczema) and children with lowered resistance are predisposed.

Clinical Findings

Local and general inflammatory signs of varying degree.

Treatment

Antibiotic therapy, possibly surgical intervention.

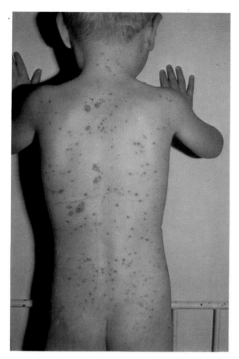

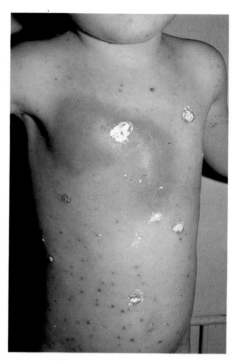

134   Three-year-old boy admitted to hospital on the tenth exanthematous day; varicella subsiding. History: agitated, severe itching and intense scratching.

135   On the same infant, extensive, inflammatory, reddened, fluctuating swelling of the anterior thoracic wall which is painful on pressure. The phlegmon has originated from a scratched varicella vesicle. Streptococcal pus is extracted on incision. Healing by antibiotic treatment.

Aphthous Stomatitis

Definition

Aphthous or herpetic stomatitis is the manifestation of primary infection with herpes simplex virus. In almost all cases, primary infection occurs during infancy. The virus remains in the organism without apparent signs and later causes recurrent herpetic diseases such as labial, genital, and corneal herpes.

Clinical Findings

Yellowish-white, painful, aphthous lesions develop from lentil-sized vesicles on the oral mucosa. The mucosa is reddened, swollen, and bleeds easily. The lesions cause increased salivation, bad breath, and regional lymphadenitis.

Treatment

Analgesic treatment by application of local anesthetics and prevention of pain by administration of soft, bland diet.

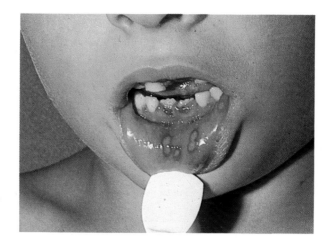

136   Aphthous stomatitis in a girl aged six years, ten months. Multiple aphthous lesions of the oral mucosa. Additional finding: typical normal indentation of permanent incisors which have just come through.

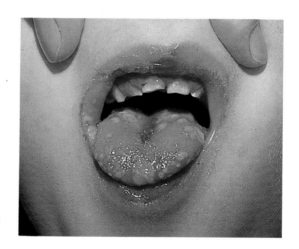

137   Aphthous stomatitis of tongue and lips.

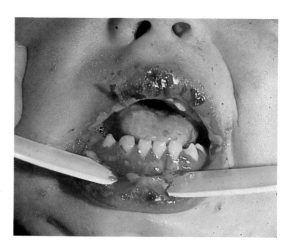

138   Severe aphthous stomatitis, partly with bleeding aphthous lesions, gingivitis, cheilitis, salivation, refusal of food, fever.

Mumps

Definition

Epidemic parotitis is a viral infection with an incubation period of 18 to 21 days. School children are predisposed; the incidence is high, 50 per cent of the infections pass without apparent signs and lifelong immunity will remain.

Clinical Findings

Painful, doughy swelling of one parotid gland appears after several days of uncharacteristic prodrome, in some cases even without any prodromal signs. In most cases, the contralateral gland will also be affected after one to two days. Other salivary glands, as well as the pancreas, may be affected simultaneously. Complicating orchitis is a rare finding. It does not appear before puberty. Concomitant abacterial meningitis is more common. It may appear during the prodrome, during or after the infection, or without any apparent parotitis. The course is benign.

Differential Diagnosis

Localization below and *in front* of the ear is an important criterion helping to differentiate parotitis from lymphadenitis of the neck which is found below and *behind* the ear. Doughy consistency of the swelling and difficulty in finding its borders by palpation are other signs to aid differentiation.

Treatment

Symptomatic.

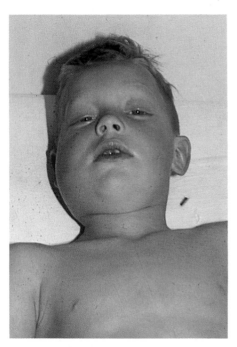

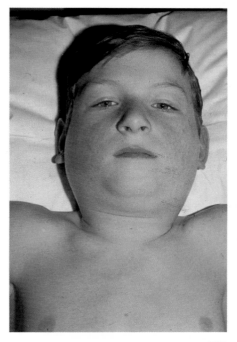

139 Four-year-old boy with right-sided epidemic parotitis and prodromal mumps meningitis. Two days before the swelling became apparent, meningitic symptoms were present with CSF pleocytosis at 4000/3 cells.

140 Mumps in a nine-year-old boy. After a meningitic prodrome lasting three days, the right-sided parotid swelling appeared one day prior to that on the left.

Poliomyelitic Facial Palsy

Definition

In one per cent of acute anterior polio-myelitis – which is a rare disease today – the poliovirus affects the anterior horn cells and motor nuclei in the brainstem. Typical flaccid paralyses with irregular distribution in the innervation areas of spinal and cerebral nerves result.

Clinical Findings

Lack of motion on the affected side of the face, lagophthalmos, and a flattened naso-labial fold indicate facial palsy, which in most cases is peripheral and also is the most common of all poliomyelitic pareses of cerebral nerves III through XI.

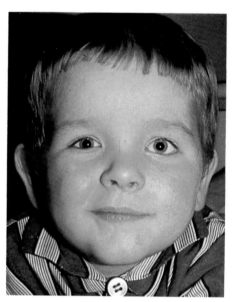

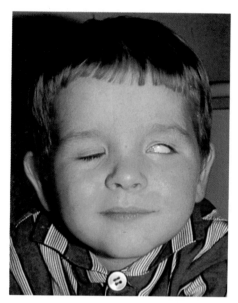

141   Left-sided facial palsy in poliomyelitis (Type III); wide palpebral fissure, smooth nasolabial fold.

LMN lesion

142   Bell's phenomenon: when trying to close the eye, the palpebral fissure stays open and the bulbus turns upwards.

Pertussis (Whooping Cough)

Definition

Pertussis is an acute infectious disease caused by *Bordetella pertussis*. The incubation period is seven to fourteen days. The disease is characterized by repeated paroxysmal coughs, passing through several stages, and lasting several weeks.

Clinical Findings

Cough during the catarrhal or prodromal stage is uncharacteristic but highly infective, becoming paroxysmal in the convulsive stage and subsiding in the convalescent stage. Coughing is characterized by a series of rapid short, convulsive, intractable coughing spells. These are followed by deep inspiration with the typical crow-like sound. Then, the next attack will follow. The tongue protrudes, the face turns red then blue, and is swollen; tears stream from the eyes. At the end of an attack, mucus may be coughed up from the bronchi and vomiting may also occur. The diagnosis is confirmed by the typical leukocytosis and lymphocytosis, by typical roentgenograms showing the picture of so-called pertussis-lung with a basal or even larger opaque triangle, by the lack of response to codeine, and by the ability to provoke coughing attacks by intravenously administered lobeline.

Differential Diagnosis

The younger the infant, the less characteristic are the signs of pertussis; they are similar to those of spastic bronchitis – the typical "whoop" is almost always absent. In mucoviscidosis there is often a pertussoid cough.

Treatment

Antibiotics and sedatives are recommended.

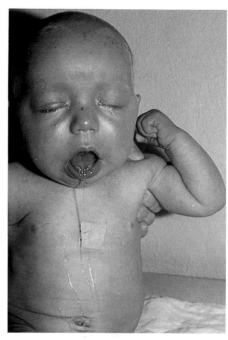

143 Four-month-old infant during a pertussis paroxysm: congestive, swollen face, lacrimation, and salivation.

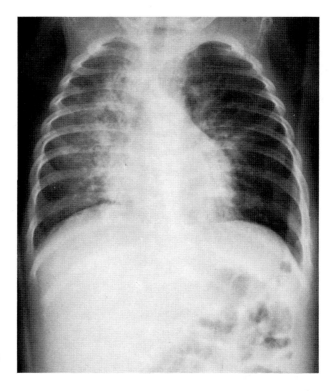

144 Central, interstitial pneumonic and peribronchitic infiltrations in pertussis during the convalescent stage. Nine-month-old infant. Complications included rachitic rosary on the roentgenogram.

β-hemolytic strep.
I mark 2-5 d

Scarlet Fever

Definition

Scarlet fever is an infectious disease of lower communicability caused by group A streptococci which, like their toxins, cause betahemolysis. Children between three and nine years of age are predisposed. The incubation period is two to five days. Antitoxic immunity is long-lasting; other streptococcal infections may occur later, but scarlet fever will not recur.

Clinical Findings

The disease starts with a sudden rise of temperature and difficulties with swallowing caused by streptococcal pharyngitis with bright red enanthem of the soft palate. Vomiting may also occur. Later, the punctate scarlatinal exanthem will follow. Signs, intensity and duration are variable. Generally, the erythema is finely papular and grouped around hair follicles with a velvety surface and slight icteric background. It is often marked in the axillary and inguinal regions. The chin and mouth are not affected (circumoral pallor). The rash fades after a few days and may be followed by branny to lamellar desquamation. During the first few days the tongue is greyish-white, after the third day of illness the typical strawberry tongue may be found. The blood count is characterized by leukocytosis and eosinophilia. A positive Rumpel-Leede sign is the manifestation of capillary damage by toxins.

Treatment

With the administration of penicillin, scarlet fever has become a harmless disease. Bacterial and toxic-allergic complications like otitis media, cervical lymphadenitis, carditis, rheumatic fever, and diffuse glomerulonephritis occur in only two to five per cent of cases today (previously 20 to 30 per cent).

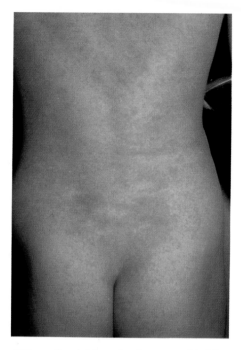

145a Scarlet fever in nine-year-old girl on third day of illness. Exanthem has been present for 24 hours. Enanthem angina, Rumpel-Leede positive. Hemolytic streptococci in throat swab.

145b Fresh scarlatinal exanthem in a 12-year-old girl. Angina lacunaris. 38.3° C. Leukocytes 25 720 m. Urobilinogenuria.

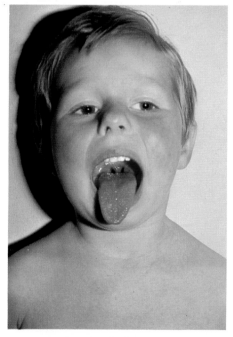

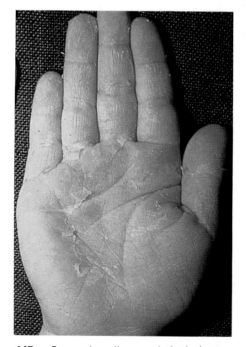

146 Scarlatinal face with circumoral pallor, strawberry tongue and infected throat, on third day of illness. Girl aged 4 years.

147 Coarse-lamellar scarlatinal desquamation of hands and feet during the second and third week of illness. Five-year-old girl.

Scarlatinal Impetigo

Definition

While in classical scarlet fever the place of entry for hemolytic streptococci is the pharyngeal lymph nodes, in scarlatinal impetigo streptococci enter the organism through skin lesions. The scarlatiniform exanthem of injured children (occurring especially after scalding in 10 per cent of the cases) is a true scarlatinal impetigo less often than believed; desquamation of skin, scarlatinal complications, and streptococci are absent. Since staphylococci are found more frequently, the toxic origin of the exanthem owing to burns or staphylococcal toxins should be considered.

Clinical Findings

Temperature rises as a scarlatiniform exanthem appears; enanthem and pharyngitis are absent, pharyngeal cultures are negative.

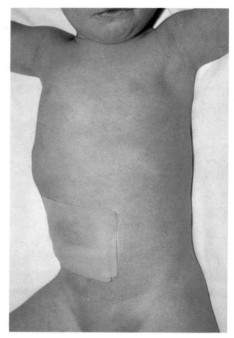

148   Scarlatinal impetigo in a 17-month-old boy five days after scalding of the abdominal skin.

Erysipelas of the Face

Definition

Erysipelas is an infectious skin disease caused by streptococci. It is rarely found today.

Clinical Findings

From the site of entry of the infective agents an erythema which rises slightly above the surface, rapidly spreads peripherally. Demarcation from normal skin is distinct. General manifestations such as fever and vomiting are also present. Formation of superficial vesicles (vesicular erysipelas) or conversion into phlegmon (phlegmonous erysipelas) may occur.

Treatment

With penicillin, the previously severe disease poses no problem.

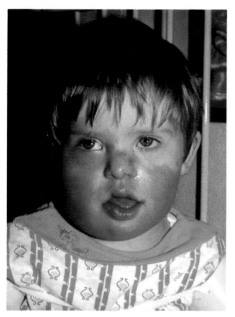

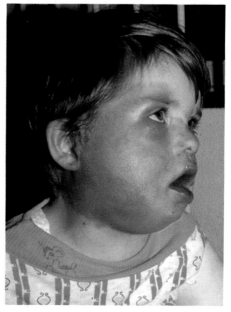

149   Facial erysipelas in a 30-month-old oligophrenic boy. Onset two days previously with high fever, swelling and redness of upper lip.

150   Typical distinct demarcation of the erythema from the surrounding normal skin. Rapid healing under treatment with penicillin.

Acute Lymphadenitis

Definition

Acute lymphadenitis is caused by infection of a regional lymph node by pyogenic germs, mainly staphylococci and streptococci. The infective agents originate from a primary inflammatory process in the supply area of the respective lymph nodes.

Clinical Findings

Pyogenic lymphadenitis is most frequently encountered in the cervical region, subsequent to tonsillitis and otitis, or even without any apparent infection. The groin is another frequent site of lymphadenitis caused by infected injuries of the leg. Local swelling, tenderness on palpation, rubor, and fluctuation appear along with elevated temperature. Red, tender lymphatics caused by lymphangitis are rarely found on extremities.

Differential Diagnosis

Specific lymphadenitis (tuberculosis, cat scratch disease) as well as noninflammatory swelling of lymph nodes (leukemia, lymphogranuloma, lymphosarcoma) have to be excluded.

Treatment

Antibiotics, puncture or incision.

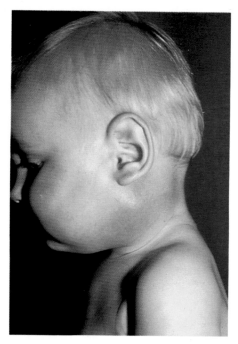

151 Lymphadenitis of the neck in a boy of 15 months. Onset of swelling three days previously. Swelling was mistaken for mumps. Pain on pressure, so far no fluctuation.

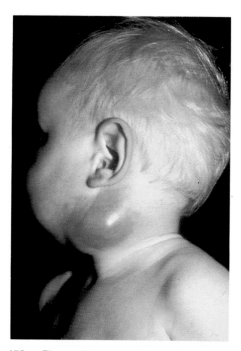

152 Fluctuation present four days later. After incision, evacuation of large amounts of pus. Bacteriologically: hemolytic streptococci.

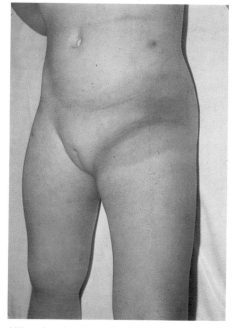

153 Inguinal lymphadenitis in a girl aged two years, eight months. Site of entry of infective agents was not found. Incision after three days found staphylococcus aureus haemolyticus in the pus.

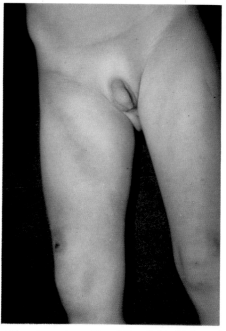

154 Lymphangitis of the right thigh and swollen inguinal lymph nodes owing to furuncle on the knee. Infective agents: hemolytic streptococci. Age of boy: four years, four months.

Phlegmon of the Floor of the Mouth

Definition

The lowered immunity of the neonate predisposes it to phlegmonous processes caused by staphylococci entering subcutaneous tissue through lesions of the skin. Scalp, the periorbital region, the floor of the mouth, and thoracic wall are sites of predilection.

Clinical Findings

Swelling and reddening of the submental region are the clinical manifestations of phlegmon of the floor of the mouth. Collateral edema expands on both sides. There is only limited impairment of drinking and swallowing; salivation is increased.

Treatment

The phlegmon will heal after incision and counteropening aided by antibiotic treatment.

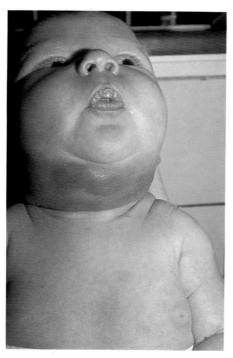

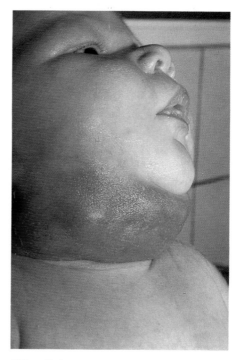

155   Phlegmon of the floor of the mouth in a twelve-day-old infant. Fever and salivation; leukocytes: 22,000 μl.

156   Rubor, swelling, and fluctuation of submental region. Healing within one week after evacuation of pus through the incision (staphylococcus aureus), drainage lasted four days and erythromycin was administered.

Septic Phlegmon

Definition

In children with lowered resistance, highly infective staphylococci and streptococci may lead to rapidly progressing, inflammatory disease of soft tissues. Death may result after a fulminant course with septic manifestations.

Clinical Findings

Under septic fever and circulatory insufficiency, expanding rubor and swelling of the skin turn into hemorrhagic necroses. The cervical region and thoracic and abdominal walls are the sites most frequently affected.

Treatment

Massive antibiotic therapy, administration of gammaglobulin, stabilization of the circulatory system.

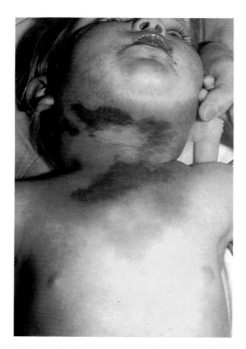 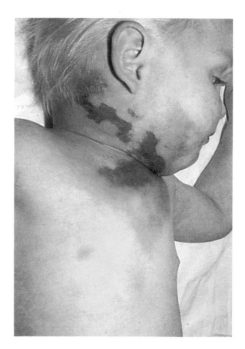

157 and 158 Extensive phlegmon of the neck with hemorrhagic necroses. Circulatory failure. Therapy-resistant, irresistible deterioration with increase in cutaneous hemorrhage in the area of the phlegmon. Fatal outcome within 19 hours.

Rheumatic and Allergic Diseases

Annular Rheumatic Erythema

Definition

Annular erythema is a transitory, allergic, cutaneous phenomenon encountered during the course of rheumatic fever in ten per cent of the cases.

Clinical Findings

Discrete, pink, round or polycyclic efflorescences appear on the trunk. There is no pruritus. The lesions disappear within a few days but may recur.

Differential Diagnosis

Different forms of erythema have to be excluded: polyetiologic erythema annulare centrifugum (Darier), rather similar erythema gyratum persistens and repens, infectious erythema, urticaria gyrata and eczema marginatum (Hebrae).

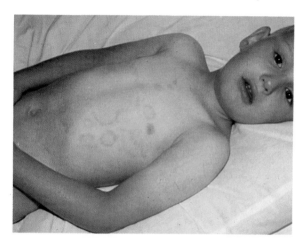

159   Rheumatic fever in a boy aged 4 years 8 months. Annular erythema on the trunk in the second week of illness.

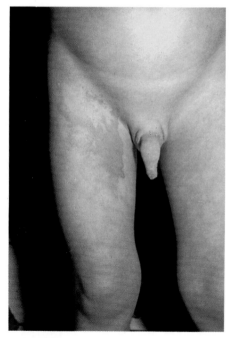

160   Three-year-old, auburn boy with erythema gyratum persistens on the thigh. Condition unchanged for 30 months. No fungi found. Histologically: capillary hemangioma.

Erythema Nodosum

Definition

Erythema nodosum (contusiform erythema) is an unspecific allergic phenomenon. It occurs frequently during childhood, but most of all in the course of primary tuberculosis with the appearance of tuberculous allergy, i.e., six to eight weeks after primary infection. It also occurs as an allergic reaction to different agents: drugs (sulfonamides), toxins (streptococci, rheumatic fever), as well as Boeck's sarcoid (Löfgren-syndrome: erythema nodosum, bilateral hilar enlargement, transient articular complaints).

Clinical Findings

On the extensor sides of the extremities there are painful infiltrations that are slightly elevated and hard on palpation. The size of the lesions ranges from that of a pea to that of a walnut; the color turns from bright red to blue. The anterior side of the lower leg is most frequently affected. The lesions disappear – often showing an intermittent, relapsing course – within two to three weeks. The presence of erythema nodosum should always initiate diagnostic measures for tuberculosis (BCG-vaccination, tuberculin tests, roentgenograms).

Differential Diagnosis

Erythema induratum Bazin never appears before puberty and occurs almost exclu-

sively in girls. It is located on the flexor side of the lower leg and is less painful and easily ulcerates.

Treatment

Therapy of the underlying disease.

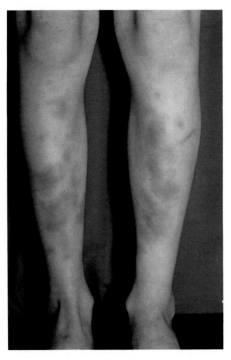

161 Erythema nodosum present for one week. Ten-yearold boy with primary tuberculosis of the lung.

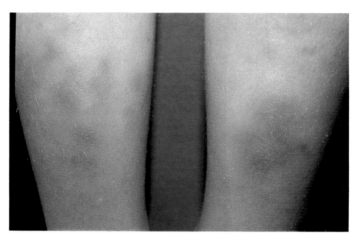

162   Recent erythema nodosum. Seven-year-old boy. Fever, ESR: 75/107, bullous positive Tine-tuberculin-test. For roentgenologic findings, see Fig. 163.

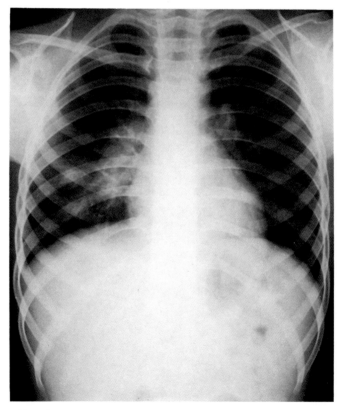

163   Chest X-ray of the patient in Fig. 162. Primary tuberculous complex in the right midlung zone (bipolar stage) with perifocal hilar infiltration.

Blood Diseases

Leukemia

Definition

Leukemia is a malignant neoplastic disease of the hematopoietic tissue as characterized by irreversible increase in the number of leukocytes. In childhood the acute form occurs almost exclusively, the highest incidence being between the third and fifth year of life. In the white blood count either undifferentiated stem cells (stem cell leukemia, 85 per cent of cases) or immature myelocytes (acute myeloid leukemia) are found. The number of cells in the peripheral blood may or may not be increased. Chronic myelogenous leukemias of the adult type occur in only two to five percent of cases. Leukemia is an intermittent, relapsing disease. So far there is no definite cure.

Clinical Findings

Anemia (pallor, fatigue, lack of appetite), swollen lymph nodes (neck, liver, spleen), increased hemorrhagic tendency (petechiae, epistaxis), and fever attacks are the main clinical signs. Blood tests show an increased sedimentation rate, normochromic anemia, granulocytopenia, thrombocytopenia and a total white blood count in stem cell leukemia of usually less than 10,000/µl (aleukemic course), in acute myeloid leukemia of between 10,000 and 20,000/µl (subleukemic form), or more than 20,000/µl (leukemic course). Bone marrow findings prove the diagnosis.

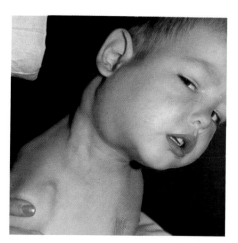

164   Cervical lymphomas in a three-year-old boy with stem cell leukemia. Swelling of lymph nodes is more common in stem cell leukemia than in acute myeloid leukemia.

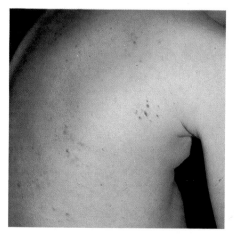

165   Disseminated, petechial, cutaneous hemorrhage in a ten-year-old girl. First recurrence of acute myelogenous leukemia. Thrombocyte count: 26,000.

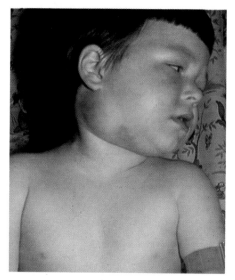

166   Classic triad of symptoms: extreme pallor, cutaneous hemorrhage, swelling of lymph nodes. Three-year-old girl with stem cell leukemia. Ecchymosis over nuchal lymphomas, petechiae on flexor surface of left elbow (Rumpel-Leede).

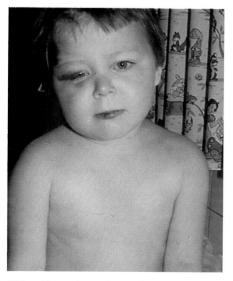

167   Five days later (child Fig. 166): extensive cranial hemorrhage, hemorrhage of the oral mucosa. Mikulicz syndrome: swelling on infiltration of the right-sided lacrimal and salivary glands. Erythrocytes: 1.9 mill./µl, Hb 5.4 g per 100 ml, thrombocytes: 5000.

Differential Diagnosis

Frequently leukemic children are admitted to the hospital under diagnoses such as anemia, recurrent lymphadenitis, hemorrhagic diathesis, or rheumatic fever.

Treatment

At the present moment, an average survival time of 18 to 30 months is attained by cytostatic and antibiotic treatment, blood transfusions, and differentiated administration of corticosteroids.

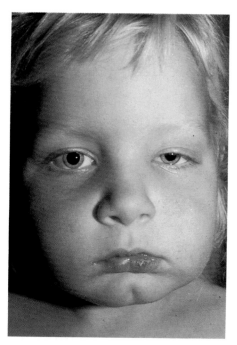

168   Mikulicz syndrome in acute stem cell leukemia. Swelling of left salivary and parotid gland. Four-year-old girl.

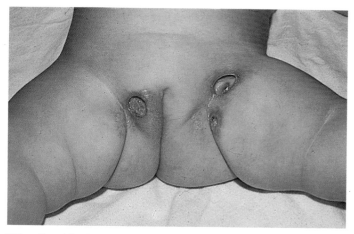

169   Torpid ulcerations in a 15-month-old girl with stem cell leukemia. The ecthyma is a manifestation of the lowered resistance and reaction of the leukemic infant.

Idiopathic Thrombocytopenic Purpura

Definition

Idiopathic thrombocytopenic purpura (Werlhof's disease) is the most common hemorrhagic diathesis of childhood. It is caused by increased destruction of platelets in the peripheral blood. This may be an acute allergic reaction one to two weeks after noxious viral effects or drug administration, or less frequently, a chronic recurrent state owing to autoantibodies.

Clinical Findings

There are bright red petechiae (fleabite hemorrhage) closely packed in irregular distribution, lentil-sized, blue-red, hemorrhagic spots in the skin, and blue patches which later turn to yellow or green subcutaneous hemorrhages. They may reach the size of a palm (leopard skin) and are mainly found on portions of the body which are exposed to pressure. Hemorrhage of the mucous membranes of nose, mouth, and eyes is frequently present. Intestinal hemorrhage is encountered less frequently and is painless in contrast to anaphylactoid purpura. The general condition of the patient is hardly affected. The Rumpel-Leede test is positive, the platelet count shows less than 50,000/µl in most of cases; bleeding and retraction time are prolonged, clotting time is normal.

Treatment

Corticosteroids are the drugs of choice.

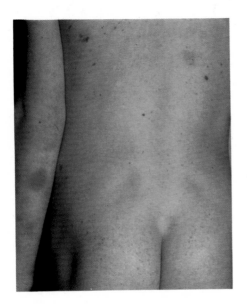

170   Ten-year-old boy with acute thrombocytopenic purpura which appeared one week after rubella infection. Note the closely set petechiae on the buttocks, lentil-sized hemorrhages on the back and subcutaneous dime-size hematomas on the lower arm. Thrombocytes: 19,000; bleeding time: 45 min; clotting time: 90.

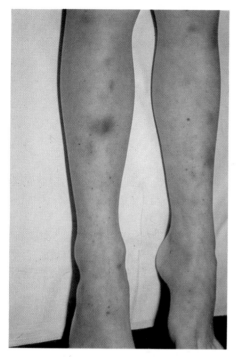

171 Pressure hematomas are more frequently found on the lower leg.

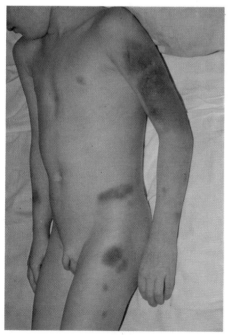

172 Ecchymoses after minor trauma. This may be mistaken for severe maltreatment.

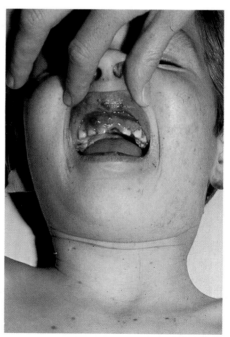

173 Besides the gingival hemorrhage, there is also hemorrhage of the buccal mucosa and the tonsils. Under treatment with corticosteroids, regression of thrombocytopenic purpura occurs within two weeks. A six-year-old sister of the child, who was also affected with Werlhof's disease two years later, is shown in Figs. 170 to 173.

Hemophilia

Definition

This blood disease is a hereditary hemorrhagic condition which is characterized by a sex-linked, recessive trait chromosome and lack of clotting factor VIII (hemophilia A, 80 per cent of the cases) or IX (hemophilia B, 20 per cent of the cases). The disease appears only in males. The rate is 1:4000. The disease is transmitted by women with normal phenotype. In 30 to 40 per cent of the cases, no familial trait is present (sporadic hemophilia).

Clinical Findings

The most striking manifestation of the disease is hemorrhage after minor trauma (hemorrhage of the gums in dentition, epistaxis) which is most difficult to stop. Especially in infants, blunt trauma will cause large cutaneous hemorrhage. Petechiae do not occur. During school age, arthrotic alterations occur owing to recurrent bleeding into the joints (hemophilic joint). Clotting time is prolonged, bleeding time is normal, thromboplastin time is normal as well, whereas recalcification time is prolonged, and the prothrombin consumption test is pathologic (more than 20 per cent). The thromboplastin generation test allows differentiation of hemophilia A from hemophilia B.

Treatment

The missing clotting factors are substituted by administration of plasma concentrates. Factor VIII may also be given by transfusion of fresh blood, factor IX by transfusion of fresh or stored blood.

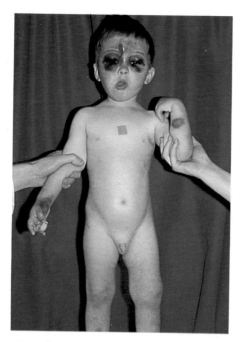

174 Two-year-old boy with hemophilia A. First cutaneous hemorrhage at the age of 5 months. Now, after a fall, extensive subcutaneous hemorrhages of face, lower arms, legs, and hemarthrosis of left knee are evident.

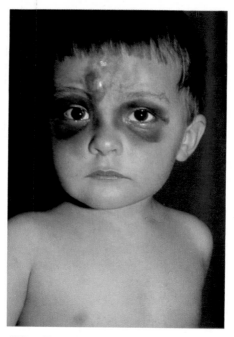

175 Frontal cephalhematoma accompanying cutaneous hemorrhage.

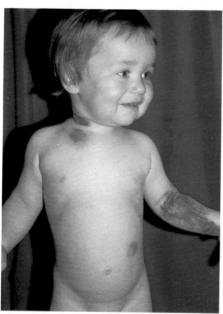

176 One-year-old boy with sporadic hemophilia A. Large patches of cutaneous hemorrhage. Hemorrhagic anemia, Hb 3.1 g per 100 ml, erythrocytes 2.73 mill./μl. Remaining activity of factor VIII 2 per cent.

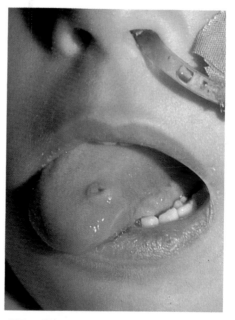

177 The boy, now five years, nine months old, almost bled to death from this small tongue bite (child of Figs. 174 and 175). Three weeks of factor VIII concentrate substitution were necessary to stop the bleeding.

Anaphylactoid Purpura

Definition

Anaphylactoid purpura (Schönlein-Henoch) is a vascular bleeding disorder caused by allergic capillary damage. Therefore, it is often found one to two weeks after some infection or after administration of some allergizing drug or food. Small infants are most frequently affected.

Clinical Findings

The hemorrhagic cutaneous lesions are pinhead to pea-sized, show a symmetrical distribution over extremities and buttocks, do not appear on the trunk, and usually originate from urticarial efflorescences (purpura urticans). Rheumatoid joint complaints (rheumatic purpura), colicky abdominal pains (abdominal purpura), and hematuria are other common findings. The intermittent, relapsing course of the disease, the favorable prognosis, and normal hematologic findings correspond to the allergic nature of the disease.

Treatment

Corticosteroids

Table 3. Differentiation of Purpuras

	Petechiae generalized	localized (extremities)	Large bruises (suffusions, ecchymoses)
Thrombopathy (Werlhof)	+		+
Vasopathy (Schönlein-H.)		+	
Coagulopathy (hemophilia)			+

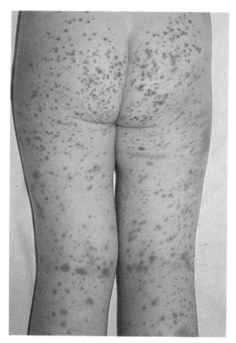

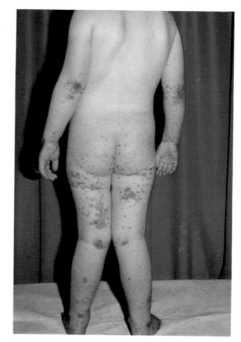

178 Rheumatic purpura in a four-year-old boy. Petechiae with symmetrical distribution appear over the buttocks and extremities. Articular swelling and pain were present.

179 Anaphylactoid purpura, 30-month-old girl. Distribution of hemorrhagic lesions is typical. Additional finding: knock-knees corresponding to age.

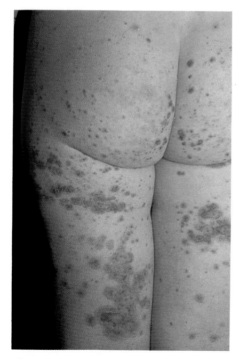

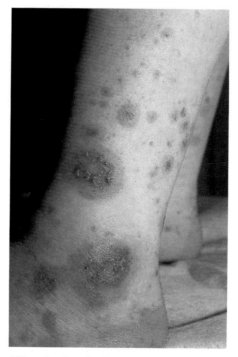

180 Pinhead to lentil-sized hemorrhagic lesions are sometimes found on an erythematous festooned base.

181 Partly raised urticarial hemorrhages.

Diseases of the Respiratory Tract

Croup

Definition

Croup or pseudocroup is an acute constricting inflammatory disease of the mucous membranes of the larynx (subglottic laryngitis, constricting laryngotracheitis). It appears mainly in small infants. There are different pathogenetic factors: allergic reactions, viral infections, air pollution, and metereologic conditions (cold, dry air).

Clinical Findings

A triad of symptoms is typical: barking cough, hoarseness and inspiratory stridor. They develop in the course of a viral infection of the upper respiratory tract. In most night cases, sudden life-threatening dyspnea may arise showing jugular and epigastric retraction, intense restlessness, and finally unconsciousness, failure of the circulatory system, and death by suffocation. Often no cyanotic stage is noticeable. If, in the threatening constricting stage, barking cough and hoarseness are replaced by painful swallowing, choked voice, and salivation, the particularly grave disease of acute epiglottitis is present (supraglottic laryngitis).

Treatment

Conservative treatment consists of administration of corticosteroids, antibiotics, and sedatives, as well as fresh air, moist air, or oxygen. In serious cases tracheostomy is required.

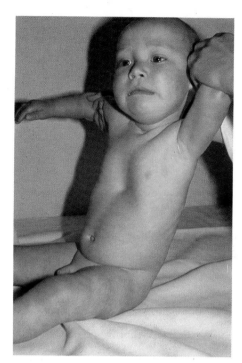

182 Eight-month-old infant with pseudo-croup: sudden onset of severe dyspnea, gasping hoarse inspirations, deep jugular and sternal retraction, livid skin, and frightened expression.

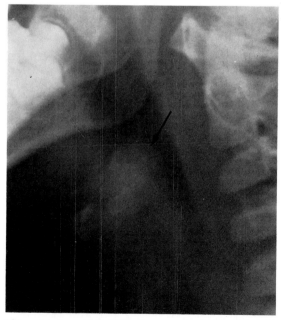

183 Acute epiglottitis in a seven-year-old girl. Although the throat was sore, there was no cough or hoarseness. There was severe inspiratory dyspnea with swelling of the epiglottis evident on roentgenograms. Tracheostomy and cure.

Diseases of the Gastrointestinal Tract

Esophageal Atresia

Definition

In congenital esophageal occlusion, the proximal portion of the esophagus ends blindly at the level of the second or third thoracic vertebra. In 90 per cent of the cases there is a fistula between the distal portion of the esophagus and the trachea (Type IIIb according to Vogt). In eight per cent of the cases there is no esophago-tracheal fistula (Type II). In the remaining rare cases, there are communications between the trachea and either the upper and lower (Type IIIc) or the upper portion only (Type IIIa). The incidence is believed to be one in 2000 births. One third of the cases is associated with prematurity and hydramnios.

Clinical Findings

Discharge of saliva and foamy mucus from the mouth of the newborn is the major clinical symptom. At the first feeding, nonacidified food is brought up immediately. Aspiration of saliva and food is indicated by dyspneic and cyanotic attacks. An inserted gastric tube meets resistance after ten to fifteen centimeters and rolls up. The diagnosis is confirmed by radiography with water-soluble contrast medium; air-filled stomach and bowel indicate lower tracheal fistula.

Treatment

The malformation can be treated successfully by surgical correction. The diagnosis must be made within the first three days of life. Without surgical intervention all affected children die from aspiration pneumonia. The general prognosis is lowered by the fact that in about one-third of the cases additional malformations (congenital heart disease, intestinal atresia) and prematurity are present.

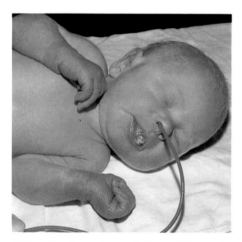

184   Esophageal atresia in a 48-hour-old newborn. Foaming at the mouth and cyanosis are typical.

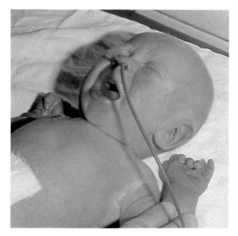

185   Blocking and bending of a rubber catheter inserted through the nose.

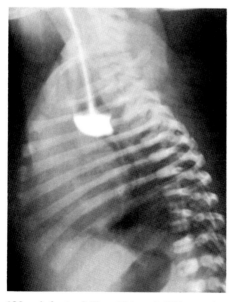

186   Infant of Figs. 184 and 185: on the roentgenogram, a blind pouch appears in the upper third of the esophagus, where the coiled catheter is visible. The stomach is filled with air. Surgical intervention: esophageal atresia type Vogt IIIb.

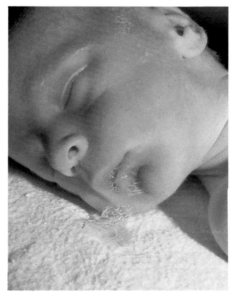

187   This aspect of the premature infant (weight 1840 g) showing foamy salivation allows the tentative diagnosis of esophageal atresia. Confirmed by roentgenograms (type IIIb), surgical intervention, fatal outcome.

Pyloric Stenosis

Definition

Pylorospasm (spastic hypertrophic pyloric stenosis) is a congenital disease of unknown origin. It becomes clinically apparent during the first six months of life. Pyloric spasticity and hypertrophy cause a characteristic obstructive syndrome. Eighty per cent of the affected children are boys.

Clinical Findings

Preictal vomiting, externally visible gastric peristalsis, oliguria, and pseudoconstipation are the prominent clinical signs. They appear at the end of the first week at the earliest, but in most cases not before the fourth week of life. Later, hematemesis, dystrophy, dehydration, and pyloric coma may follow. Lack of gas in the small bowel, gastrectasis, delayed gastric emptying as well as narrowing and elongation of the intestinal canal are found by radiography.

Differential Diagnosis

Most of all, congenital duodenal stenosis, hiatal hernia, and the adrenogenital salt-losing defect (pseudopylorospasm) must be excluded.

Treatment

Surgical intervention by pylorotomy (Weber-Ramstedt) is indicated if conservative measures such as administration of sedatives, parasympatholytic drugs, frequent feeding, and experienced, gentle care fail to produce weight gain.

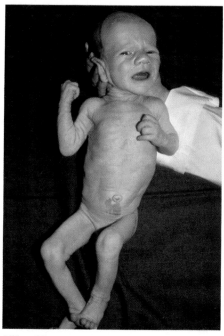

188 Three-week-old, dystrophic male with pyloric stenosis. Note the absence of subcutaneous fat, wrinkled skin and senile expression. Weight 2500 g, birth weight 2800 g. Surgical treatment.

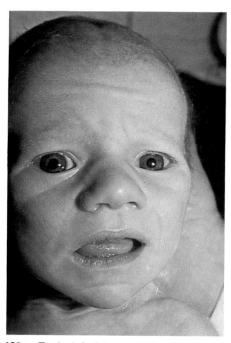

189 Typical facial expression in pyloric stenosis: wrinkled fore head, big eyes, painful mimicry, dystrophy. Three weeks old.

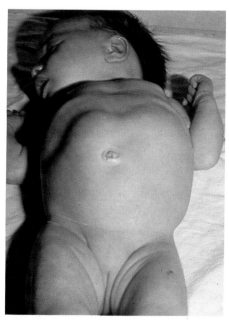

190 Typical gastric cramps in pyloric stenosis. Age four weeks. Cure by conservative treatment.

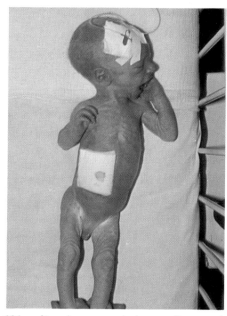

191 Atrophy caused by undiagnosed pyloric stenosis. Age six weeks, weight 2150 g, 1000 g less than birth weight. Note wasting of subcutaneous fatty tissue, the prominent ribs and pelvic bones, the wrinkled femoral skin, and senile face.

Congenital Atresia of Small Intestine

Definition

Complete congenital occlusion of the intestinal lumen is most frequently found in the rectum, the anal region, ileum, and duodenum. The incidence is about 1/3000. An occluding membrane, a solid cord of connective tissue, or localized aplasia of the respective intestinal portion may be present. In 20 per cent of the cases, intestinal obstructions are found at several sites. Atresias of the colon and small bowel do not appear simultaneously. One third of the cases of small bowel atresia are found in premature infants.

Clinical Findings

All newborns with intestinal atresia show the clinical signs of the obstructive syndrome. With a more distal localization of the block, the signs appear later. Presence of bile in the vomitus is the major sign. It appears early in duodenal atresia, which in 95 per cent of the cases is situated distally to the duodenal papilla. The middle and lower abdominal walls are retracted; discharge of meconium may appear normal. If the occlusion is situated on a lower level there will be abdominal distension, bilious vomitus, and absent or insufficient discharge of meconium. The color of the latter is atypically light. Roentgenograms of the abdomen show a typical distribution of gas-filled and gas-free portions of the bowel as well as fluid levels, thus offering valuable information as to the site of obstruction. The incidence of hydramnios increases the higher the level of gastrointestinal atresia (esophageal, duodenal atresia).

Differential Diagnosis

Aside from congenital intestinal atresia, the most important causes of intestinal obstruction in the newborn are malrotation, volvulus, Hirschsprung's disease, and meconium ileus. They all show about the same incidence.

Treatment

Immediate treatment by a pediatric surgeon.

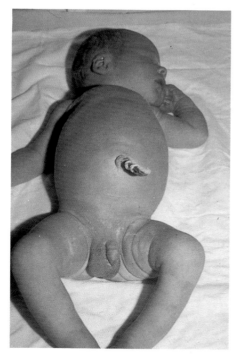

192   Atresia of the ileum, age three days.
Distended abdomen.

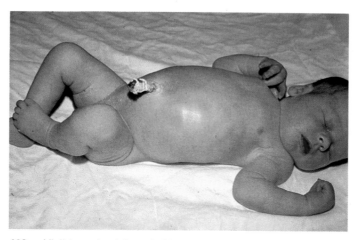

193   Visible peristalsis and shiny abdominal walls in the presence
of meteorism.

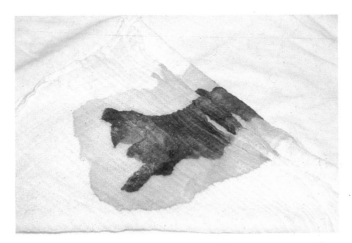

194   Bilious-fecal vomitus three days after birth in the infant shown in Figs. 192 and 193.

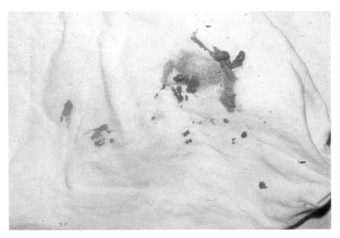

195   Repeated discharge of rubbery, light-colored intestinal contents of soft consistency. Reddish brick-dust sediment appears in the diaper.

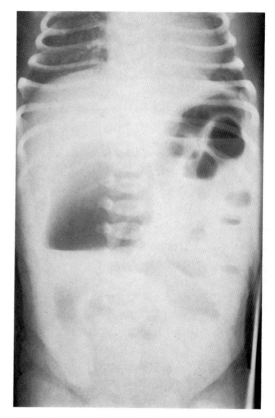

196   Several distended intestinal loops in the left upper abdomen and severely distended prestenotic loop of small bowel with fluid levels in the right middle abdomen. Surgical intervention: membranous occlusion of the distal ileum (infant in Figs. 192 to 195).

Mucoviscidosis

Definition

Mucoviscidosis (cystic fibrosis) is an autosomal-recessive hereditary disease. It manifests itself by functional disturbances of exocrine glands, hyperviscosity of secretions, obstruction of excretory ducts, and cystic fibrotic degeneration of the pancreas and lungs in particular. Morbidity is one in 1250 newborns.

Clinical Findings

In 10 per cent of the cases, the disease becomes evident by meconium ileus in the newborn period. Intestinal passage is rendered impossible by inspissated meconium in the terminal ileum. Signs of digestive insufficiency caused by lack of pancreatic enzymes appear after a few weeks, often in connection with weaning: dyspepsia, steatorrhea, meteorism, prolapse of the rectum, and dystrophy, in spite of normal appetite. At the same time, pulmonary symptoms appear with chronic recurrent bronchitis, and obstinate, afebrile, dry cough as an early sign. The diagnosis is confirmed by increased content of sodium and chloride in sweat. Values exceeding 60 mEq/l are certain proof of mucoviscidosis. Early diagnosis in the newborn is feasible by the albustix test, showing an increased content of albumin in meconium.

Differential Diagnosis

All forms of chronic growth retardation and intestinal disorders as well as chronic recurrent diseases of the respiratory organs, particularly spastic bronchitis and pertussis, must be excluded.

Treatment

A combination of therapeutic measures may help to prolong life expectancy over childhood: administration of enzymes, liquefaction of bronchial mucus, and prevention of infections.

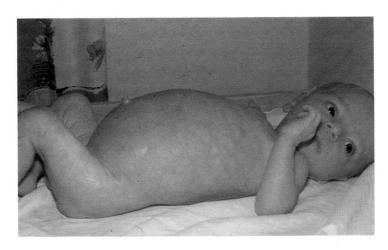

197 Mucoviscidotic infant, aged 5 months, with abdominal distention and pallor.

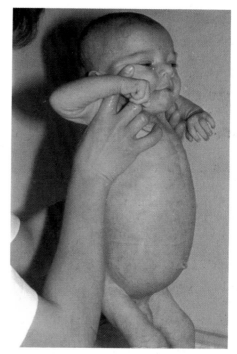

198   Dystrophy. Weight 5500 g. Birth weight 4000 g.

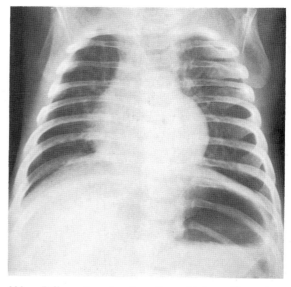

199   Diffuse, increased peribronchial markings, low diaphragm on X-ray (infant Figs. 197 and 198).

Congenital Obstruction of Bile Ducts

Definition

Congenital malformations of extrahepatic bile ducts may show complete or partial atresia, hypoplasia or stenosis. Atresia of intrahepatic bile ducts is a rare disorder. Clinically, all forms cause obstructive jaundice.

Clinical Findings

Jaundice, appearing in the second week of life, is the main clinical sign. The degree of jaundice increases subsequently, manifested by acholic stools, dark-brown urine, and progressing enlargement of the liver. Biliary cirrhosis of the liver, with hepatosplenomegaly and ascites develops after the first three months. It is followed by hepatic coma and death.

Differential Diagnosis

Obstructive jaundice may be simulated by functional disorders, such as inspissated bile after hemolytic disease of the newborn or hyperbilirubinemia of the premature infant (inspissated bile syndrome). Jaundice arising during the first 24 hours of life is always pathologic and in most cases caused by hemolytic disease of the newborn. Physiologic jaundice of the newborn generally occurs on the third or second day of life at the earliest. Sepsis (umbilical infection, osteomyelitis, meningitis), lues, hepatitis, congenital hemolytic anemia, toxoplasmosis, listeriosis, and cytomegalic inclusion disease are other possible, but less common, causes of jaundice in the neonatal period.

Treatment

The anatomical situation is explored by laparotomy. This should be done within the first three months of life. Unfortunately, surgical correction is possible in only 20 per cent of the cases.

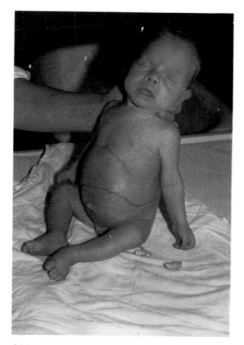 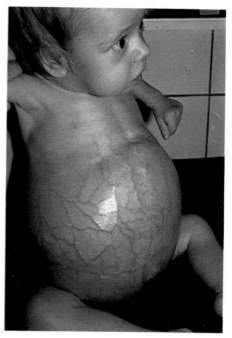

200 a and b   Intra and extrahepatic atresia of bile ducts. Age three months. Biliverdin icterus, light-colored stools, and hepatosplenomegaly were manifestations. Death occurred at the age of four months in hepatic coma.

Cutaneous Umbilicus

Definition

Cutaneous umbilicus is a harmless anomaly. Abdominal skin spreads cylindrically over the cord and is important because it is frequently mistaken for umbilical hernia with subsequent unnecessary treatment.

Clinical Findings

Cylindrical exomphalos, covered with skin, is found in place of the umbilical fossa.

Differential Diagnosis

Palpation helps to avoid the false diagnosis of umbilical hernia. In cutaneous umbilicus there is no hernial orifice except for the narrow umbilical ring.

Treatment

Not necessary. Often exomphalos will shrink and later disappearing in the abdominal fat. Thus, the cosmetic problem is also solved.

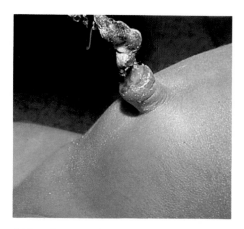

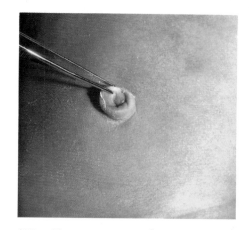

201   Cutaneous umbilicus in six-day-old infant.

202   The cutaneous umbilicus unfolds when lifted up. Additional finding: two BCG scars on the left thigh.

Umbilical Hernia

Definition

Umbilical hernia results from widening and protrusion of the umbilical scar through the umbilical ring which was closed incompletely or expanded subsequently. Increased intraabdominal pressure favors the development of the disorder (crying in neuropathy, straining in constipation, cough in pertussis). Flaccid abdominal walls also help to produce umbilical hernia (premature infants, dystrophy). Smaller hernias up to pea-size often contain only the peritoneal hernial sac. Those of cherry to walnut-size may also contain omentum and small intestine. The incidence in girls is twice that in boys.

Clinical Findings

When the infant strains or cries, a firm elastic mass protrudes over the umbilical ring. In all cases it is easily reducible. Incarceration does not occur. Palpation with the tip of the finger reveals the umbilical ring which often does not exceed five millimeters in diameter. Spontaneous tenderness or painful palpation (about five percent of the cases) indicate omental adhesions.

Treatment

Most umbilical hernias will heal spontaneously, but healing can be aided by adhesive bandages during the first year of life. Spontaneous healing is aided by regression of physiologic diastasis of the abdominal recti muscles. The muscles are strengthened by sitting and standing. If spontaneous healing fails to occur, surgical repair is done at the beginning of the second year of life.

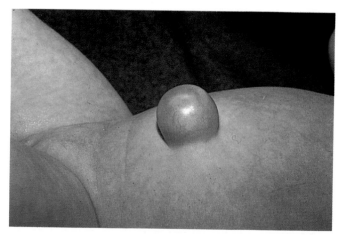

203 Cherry-sized umbilical hernia covered with thin skin of brownish discoloration. The content of the hernial sac is reducible, giving a grumbling sound. The hernial orifice may be entered by the tip of the index finger. Surgical correction was necessary in the fourth month of life, after deterioration in spite of bandaging.

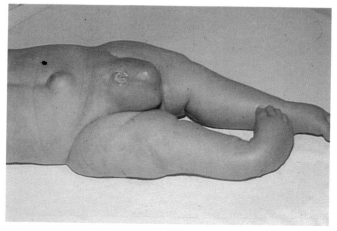

204 Umbilical and bilateral inguinal hernia (scrotal hernia) in lumbosacral myelomeningocele causing paralysis of the pelvic floor and neurogenic equinovarus. Three-month-old infant.

Supraumbilical Hernia

Definition

In supra or paraumbilical hernia, a true peritoneal hernial sac or a preperitoneal lipoma pass through a fascial defect within the linea alba directly above the umbilicus.

Clinical Findings

Directly above the umbilicus there is a protruding mass which increases in size with straining. Palpation reveals a semilunar defect within the linea alba with distinct borderlines. Peritoneal traction and omental adhesions may cause abdominal discomfort.

Treatment

Surgery.

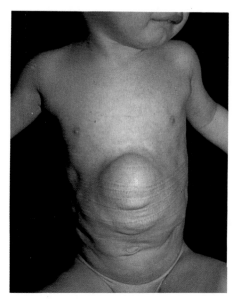

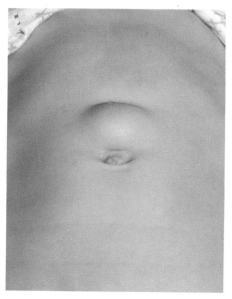

205 Supraumbilical hernia in a girl aged 20 months. No complaints.

206 The size of the supraumbilical hernia increased on abdominal pressure (crying).

Inguinal Hernia

Definition

Almost every inguinal hernia in infants or children is a congenital indirect hernia. The hernial orifice is formed by the inguinal canal. In boys the disorder is caused by failure of the processus vaginalis accompanying the spermatic cord to obliterate, in girls it results from Nuck's diverticulum following the round ligament. The general incidence is three to five per cent, 90 per cent of the affected children are boys. Sixty per cent of the hernias appear on the right side, 30 per cent on the left, and 10 per cent are bilateral.

Clinical Findings

Although a congenital defect, inguinal hernia will not appear until a few weeks after delivery in most cases. There is an increased incidence in premature and dystrophic infants and those who cry and cough a lot. The hernial sac may reach down into the scrotum (hernia vaginalis testicularis, scrotal hernia). The testicle is not palpable and overexpansion of the skin makes normal scrotal creases disappear. In some cases the scrotum completely overlaps the penis. The hernial sac may also end on a higher level along the spermatic cord (hernia vaginalis funicularis). In this case the hernia appears as a small bulge of about 2 cm diameter in front of the external inguinal ring. Incarceration threatens only during the first two years of life. In the case of a wide hernial orifice the danger is considerably lowered.

Differential Diagnosis

Firm elasticity on palpation differentiates hydrocele of the spermatic cord and testicular hydrocele from an inguinal hernia. Homogeneous transparency and dull percussion sound also aid the differential diagnosis. In most of cases, hydrocele cannot be squeezed out, while a non-strangulated hernia is reduced with a grumbling sound.

Treatment

Spontaneous healing by late obliteration of the processus vaginalis peritonei will often occur during the first year of life. In familiar affliction the prospects are reduced (30 per cent of cases). Surgical intervention is indicated in cases of strangulation, increasing size, and persistence of the disorder beyond the first year of life.

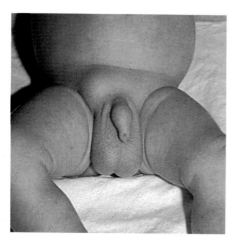

207   Right-sided funicular hernia. Eight-week-old premature twin (birth weight 1970 g).

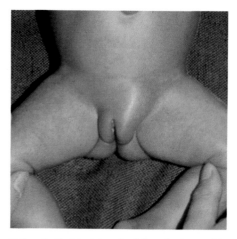

208   Left-sided inguinal hernia in an 11-week-old premature infant. Herniotomy was indicated because the ovary was within the hernial sac.

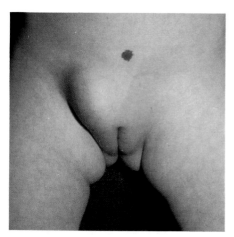

209   Right-sided walnut-sized inguinal hernia in an 18-month-old girl.

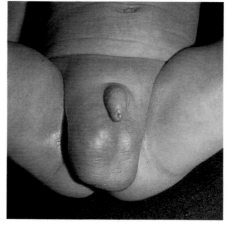

210   Large, right-sided scrotal hernia. The whole scrotum is enlarged by the enormous hernial swelling which simulates bilateral hernia. Six-month-old premature infant.

Periproctitic Abscess

Definition

Infection of the loose periproctitic tissue with subsequent suppuration may be caused by congenital perianal fistula or anal fissure secondary to injury of the anal mucosa by insertion of the thermometer, application of suppositories, scratching in oxyuriasis, or hard scybala.

Clinical Findings

Painful defecation and discharge of mucus from the anus indicate periproctitis. A painful fluctuating bulge beside the anus is the local manifestation of the disorder.

Treatment

Incision of the abscess is followed by immediate relief. Recurrence of the affection may indicate causal or secondary anal fistula demanding radical excision.

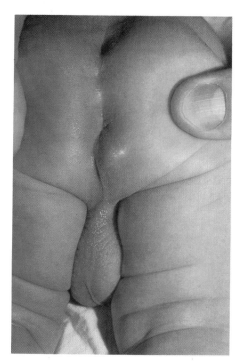

211   Periproctitic abscess in a two-month-old infant.

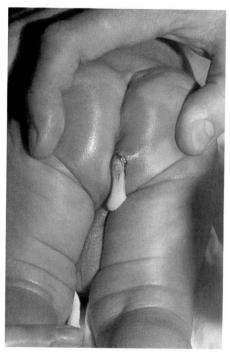

212   Coli-containing pus was removed by puncture-incision. Four relapses occurred within four weeks. Permanent cure after excision of a perianal fistula.

Diseases of Kidneys, Urinary Tract, and Genital Organs

Acute Glomerulonephritis

Definition

Acute glomerulonephritis is a postinfectious, abacterial, hematogenous, bilateral, diffuse inflammation of the glomerular capillaries. It often appears one to three weeks after a streptococcal infection of the upper respiratory tract (beta hemolytic streptococci group A, Types 1, 4, 12, and 49). Children beyond the third year of life, especially schoolchildren, are predisposed. Increase in glomerular endothelial and epithelial cells (proliferative glomerulonephritis) as well as changes in the glomerular basal membrane (membranous glomerulonephritis) are the principal morphologic manifestations.

Clinical Findings

Macro or microhematuria, edema, oliguria, hypertension, and proteinuria are the cardinal clinical findings. Proteinuria is the major symptom in predominantly membranous glomerulonephritis (nephritis with nephrotic component).

Treatment

Treatment is based on bed rest, low sodium diet, and administration of penicillin.

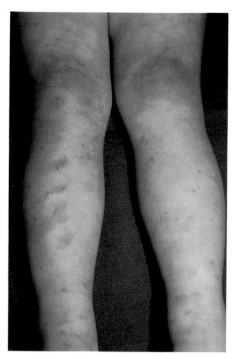

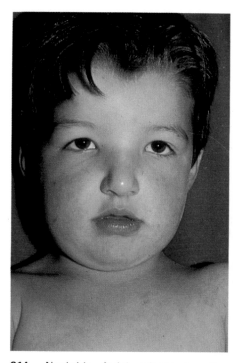

213   Pitting pretibial edema on the right side in nephritis with nephrotic tendency. Girl aged 4 years.

214   Nephritic facial edema is often discreet. As in this case, it is best recognized in the loose periorbital tissue (child of previous Fig.).

Nephrotic Syndrome

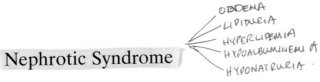

OEDEMA
LIPIDURIA
HYPERLIPEMIA
HYPOALBUMINEMIA
HYPONATRURIA .

Definition

Nephrotic syndrome is a term which comprises several disorders of different etiology, including proteinuria, hypo and dysproteinemia, edema, and hyperlipemia. Changes of the glomerular basal membrane are the underlying factors of pathologic anatomy. In lipoid nephrosis (genuine nephrosis) of small infants, this can only be proved by electron micrographs demonstrating thickening of the basal membrane. In nephritis with nephrotic component during school age, light microscopy will demonstrate predominantly membranous glomerulonephritis.

Clinical Findings

Massive generalized edema, excessive albuminuria (Esbach above 10⁰/₀₀) hypalbuminosis, hypogammaglobulinemia, hyperglobulinemia, and hypercholesterolemia exceeding 3000 mg per 100 ml, are the clinical signs of lipoid nephrosis. Hematuria, hypertension, and retention of substances normally contained in the urine are absent in pure lipoid nephrosis but will be present in mixed nephrotic-nephritic forms.

Treatment

Prednisone is the best therapeutic agent. Mixed nephrotic-nephritic forms are less responsive to prednisone. If this treatment proves unsuccessful, administration of immunosuppressive agents is indicated.

MINIMAL LESION G.N.
- yng children / adults.
- ↑ permeability of B.M => selective proteinuria ∴ hypoproteinemia + thus ↑oedema
- LIGHT μscopy => ⊘
- e⁻ μscopy => fusion of epithelial cell foot processes;
- no Ig deposition.
- accounts for 80% of cases of nephrotic syndrome
- prognosis => excellent   - 85% steroid responsive in children (60% in adults
                              - 10% steroid dependent } may need cyclophosphamide
                              - 50% steroid resistance } Rx as an adjunct

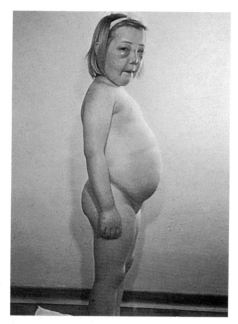

215 Ten-year-old girl with lipoid nephrosis. Marked edema, ascites.

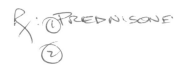

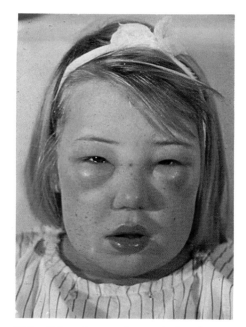

216 Edematous, distorted face. Eyes almost completely closed by swelling.

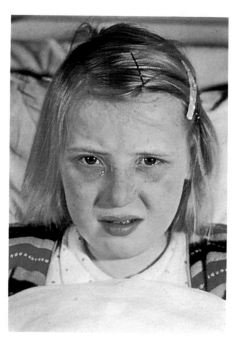

217 Edema has disappeared completely after 12 days of corticosteroid therapy. Weight loss: 12.4 kg (child of Figs. 215 and 216).

Cystic Kidney

Definition

There are different forms of congenital cystic malformations of the kidney (Figs. 218–220):
a) Hereditary, infantile, bilateral, polycystic-microcystic forms (polycystic degeneration of kidney). The prognosis is unfavorable. Death usually occurs from renal insufficiency after birth. In about five per cent of the cases cystic changes are found also in liver, spleen, pancreas, gonads, and brain. (AUTOS. RECESSIVE)
b) Hereditary, bilateral, polycystic-macrocystic forms. Survival up to adult age is possible depending on the extent of normal renal tissue present. (AUTO. DOM.)
c) Unilateral, polycystic, aplastic forms. In place of one kidney there is a conglomerate of larger and smaller cysts. Favorable prognosis after extirpation.

d) Multilocular renal cyst: favorable prognosis after surgery.
e) Solitary renal cyst: surgery depending on size, favorable prognosis.

Clinical Findings

Distended abdomen and enlarged kidneys with nodular surface on palpation are the main clinical signs. Additionally, intestinal compression with vomiting and decreased diaphragmatic movement with dyspnea may be present. Urinalysis and intravenous urography give further information.

Treatment

In unilateral forms surgery is the treatment of choice. In bilateral forms there is no treatment.

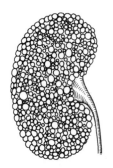 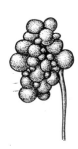 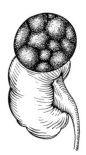 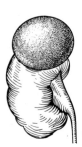

218   Forms of congenital cystic kidney (according to Grob) a) and b) polycystic renal degeneration, c) aplastic cystic kidney, d) multilocular renal cyst, e) solitary renal cyst.

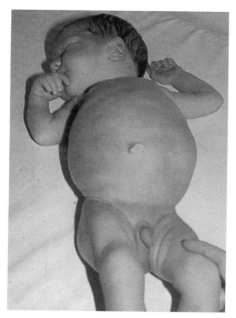

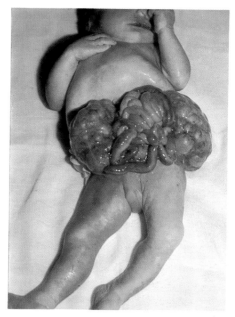

219   Left-sided dysplastic cystic kidney. Two-week-old infant. Large, distended abdomen particularly on the left side.

221   Bilateral macrocystic renal degeneration in a premature infant with a birth weight of 1750 g. Large abdomen. Death from central respiratory failure within the first few hours of life.

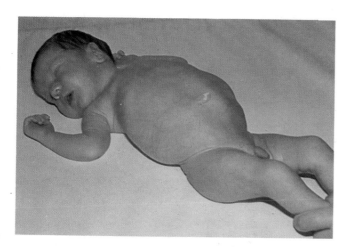

220   On palpation an egg-sized firm, nodular tumor in the left midabdomen is felt (infant Fig. 219). Urinalysis normal. Nonfunctional left kidney on pyelogram. Cure after extirpation of the aplastic cystic kidney.

Disturbed Micturition

Definition

Congenitally disturbed micturition is the result of infravesicular anatomical obstacles. These may be malformations such as constricted neck of the bladder (Marion), urethral valves, and urethral stenosis. Dilatation and infection of the bladder and supravesical urinary tract will result with subsequent damage of renal parenchyma and function.

Clinical Findings

Disturbed micturition, residual urine, urinary tract infection, and possibly a distended abdomen. The diagnosis is confirmed by cystourethrography.

Treatment

Early surgical intervention.

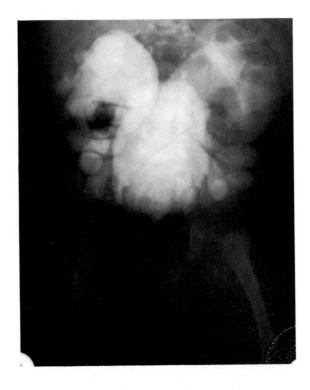

222 Extreme bilateral enlargement of renal calyces, ureters and bladder owing to urethral stenosis. Four-week-old male infant distended abdomen and paradoxical ischuria after delivery.

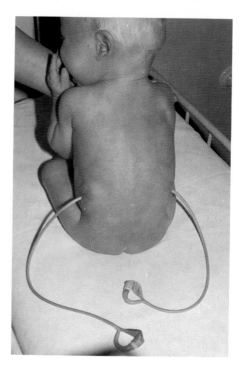

223 Bilateral nephrostomy, which is kept functioning for 18 months in order to ease tension and to allow recovery of the dilated renal pelves.

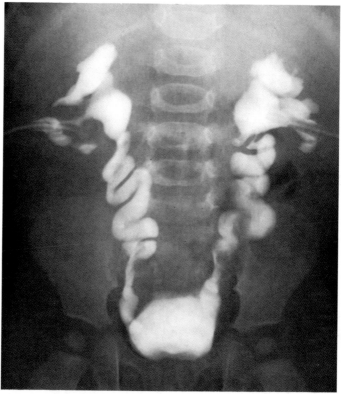

224 Urography through the two permanent catheters at the age of 16 months. Decreasing enlargement of the upper urinary tract was observed. Functional and anatomical improvement after bilateral ureteroneocystostomy and surgical correction of the urethral stenosis.

Wilm's Tumor

Definition

Wilm's tumor is a malignant, mixed embryonic tumor of the infantile kidney (nephroblastoma). Beside neuroblastoma, it is the most frequent abdominal tumor of infancy.

Clinical Findings

In most cases Wilm's tumor is not suspected until abdominal distention is visible. On careful palpation a large, painless, abdominal mass with a smooth or nodular surface is revealed. Urinary analysis shows microhematuria; on intravenous urograms, deformation or displacement of the renal pelvis is present, or cannot be visualized at all.

Differential Diagnosis

For the differential diagnosis neuroblastoma, retroperitoneal teratoma, reticulosarcoma, ovarian tumors, mesenterial cysts, cystic kidney, and hydronephrosis must be considered.

Treatment

Immediate nephrectomy combined with cytostatic treatment and roentgen radiation are necessary. Nevertheless, 60 per cent of the children will die within eighteen months of surgery owing to the high incidence of local recurrence and pulmonary metastases.

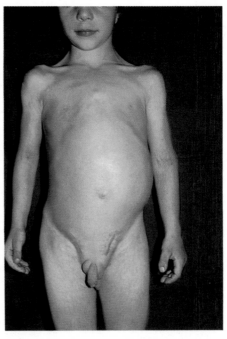

225   Wilm's tumor of the left kidney. Boy aged five years. Urinalysis normal, ESR 110/128.

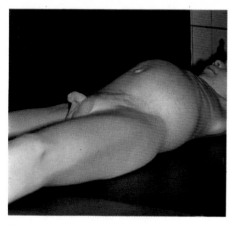

226 Considerably protruding left abdomen in the child shown in Fig. 225.

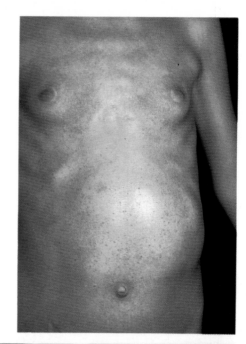

227 Eleven-year-old girl. Wilm's tumor, the size of a child's head, in left upper and middle abdomen; surface of tumor is nodular. ESR 51/88.

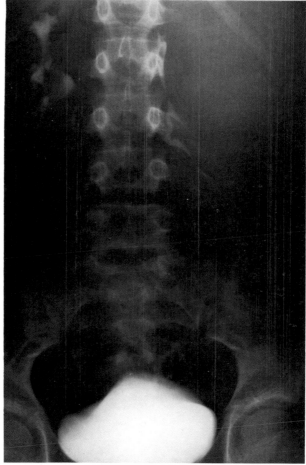

228 Infusion pyelography shows medial displacement of renal calyces by the large tumor in the left abdomen.

Hydrocele

Definition

Faulty obliteration of the processus vaginalis peritonei may cause abnormal accumulation of fluid in the tunica vaginalis
which surrounds testicle and spermatic
cord: hydrocele of spermatic cord or testes.
This harmless disorder may be congenital or
appear during the first years of life owing to
spontaneous exudation. In the newborn the
incidence is two to three per cent. About 50
per cent of hydroceles are on the right side,
20 per cent on the left; 30 per cent are bilateral.

Clinical Findings

Hydrocele appears as a painless swelling of
the scrotum or spermatic cord. It has a
firm-elastic consistency and it may vary in
size. Homogeneous transparency, discount-
ing the posterior, distal testicular shadow, is
a characteristic sign which can be demonstrated by transillumination. In some cases,
hydrocele communicates with the abdominal cavity (communicating hydrocele). In
this case it can be squeezed out. Hydrocele
of the spermatic cord has sharp ends of the
upper and lower part. This can be felt on
palpation.

Differential Diagnosis

The important differentiation from incar-
cerated inguinal hernia is facilitated by the
following characteristics of hydrocele:
homogeneous translucency, local painless-
ness, and undisturbed general condition. In
a considerable number of cases, hydrocele
and inguinal hernia appear simultaneously.

Treatment

In infants, hydrocele undergoes spontaneous regression in 90 per cent of cases. Surgical intervention is indicated after the first
year of life, particularly if inguinal hernia is
present at the same time.

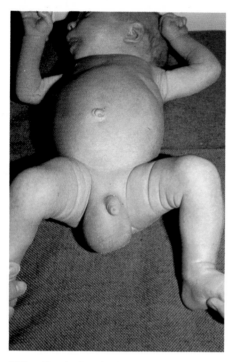

229 Testicular hydrocele of the right side. Six-week-old premature twin.

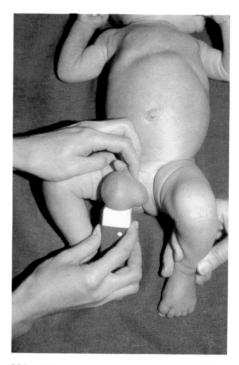

230 Homogeneous translucency. The scrotum has a firm elasticity; the testicle is not palpable.

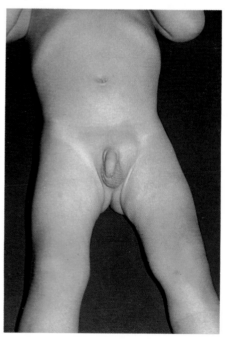

231 Hydrocele of the left spermatic cord in an 18-month-old boy. A displaceable but not reducible swelling which was not painful on pressure appeared suddenly. Spontaneous regression occurred within three months.

Balanitis

Definition

Decomposition of smegma occurring with a narrow prepuce, true phimosis, or insufficient cleansing causes inflammations of glans and prepuce in infants.

Clinical Findings

Purulent discharge from prepuce, which shows inflammatory rubor and edematous swelling. The painful disorder causes dysuria.

Treatment

Prepuce is cleaned with boric acid or potassium permanganate solution.

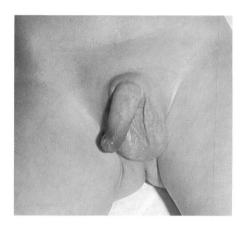

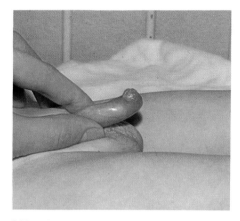

232   Trunk-like prepuce with balanitis in a boy aged two years.

233   Preputial orifice almost completely closed by swelling. Purulent discharge. Healing occurred within four days after irrigations and treatment with ointments (child in Fig. 232).

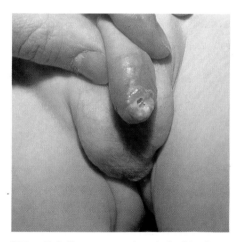

234   Febrile suppurative balanitis in a four-year-old boy. Enterococci and streptococci were found. Prepuce completely retractable after inflammation subsided; no phimosis.

Paraphimosis

Definition

Strangulation of the glans caused by retraction of the prepuce and fixation in the coronary sulcus is called paraphimosis. It appears after attempted dilatation of the prepuce or after freeing adhesions.

Clinical Findings

Strangulation causes disturbance of venous return and painful swelling of prepuce and glans or even inflammation and ulceration in case of longer duration.

Treatment

Most cases of paraphimosis can be reduced under general anesthesia without surgical intervention. If not, the dorsal portion of the preputial ring is divided over a grooved director.

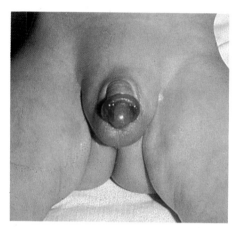

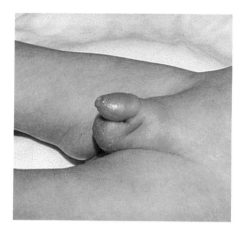

235 Paraphimosis after division of preputial adhesions in a seven-month-old infant. Note erosions of the preputial mucosa.

236 Condition immediately after manual reduction.

Hypospadias

Definition

Congenital displacement of the external urethral orifice in the proximal and lower portion of the atretic navicular fossa is called hypospadias. Depending on the position of the external orifice, there is hypospadias of the glans (in the coronary sulcus, 40 to 50 per cent of the cases), of the penis (25 to 30 per cent), and scrotal or perineal hypospadias. Simultaneously, the penis shows a hooklike deformation. The incidence is seven in 1000 male newborns.

Clinical Findings

Often, the dislocated orifice is stenosed, thus impairing micturition. In severe deformity of the penis, the urinary stream is directed backwards, forcing the boy to urinate in a sitting position. Later, there are difficulties in coitus and disturbances in fertility.

Differential Diagnosis

Together with hermaphroditic external genital organs, hypospadias may present as male or female pseudohermaphroditism. The differentiation is made by cytologic examination.

Treatment

Stenosis of the orifice has to be dilated immediately. Surgical correction of penis deformation with subsequent urethroplasty is performed before school age.

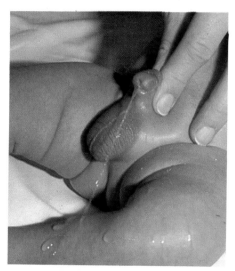

237 Hypospadias of the glans in a four-month-old premature twin. Urethral orifice is beneath the fossa navicularis on the right. Urinary stream is directed caudally.

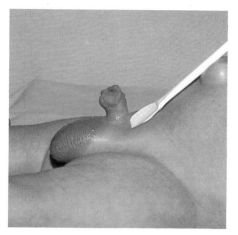

238 Hooklike penile deformation with a dorsal preputial "apron". An umbilical hernia was also found. The other twin also showed hypospadias.

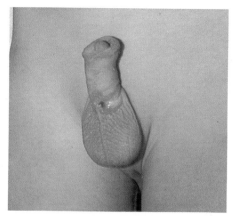

239 Hypospadias after surgical extension of penis. The urethral orifice, now situated at the root of the penis, will be displaced distally by another operation (urethroplasty).

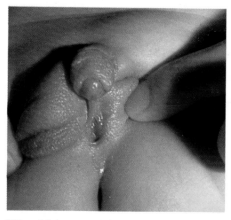

240 Male pseudohermaphroditism with intersexual external genital organs and perineo-scrotal hypospadias. Gonads are present in the divided scrotum which resemble labia. Nuclear sex: chromatin negative. Chromosomal analysis: male karyotype (XY); no mosaic (XO/XY); no structural anomaly of Y-chromosome (Prof. Pfeiffer, Münster).

Diseases of Bones and Joints

Chondrodystrophy

Definition

Chondrodystrophy (achondroplasia) is a dominant hereditary disease of mainly sporadic occurrence. It results from disturbances of endochondral ossification and causes disproportionate dwarfism. The incidence is 1 to 2/100,000.

Clinical Findings

Unproportioned growth retardation owing to shortened limbs, large skull, saddle nose, frog belly, lumbar lordosis, and waddling gait are the most striking symptoms. In serious cases, the alterations are already present at birth, in milder forms less severe changes appear later (chondrohypoplasia). Intellectual development is not affected.

Treatment

There is no treatment.

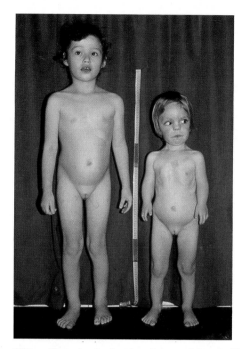

241 Chondrodystrophy in a girl aged four years, four months compared to normal child of the same age. Body length 88 cm (normally 106 cm), birth length 44 cm, micromelia of the upper extremities. The fingertips reach down to the hip joints, whereas in a normal child they reach to the midfemur.

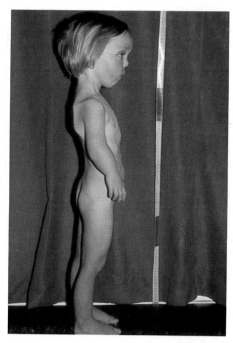

242 Large skull, saddle nose, relatively long trunk, short arms.

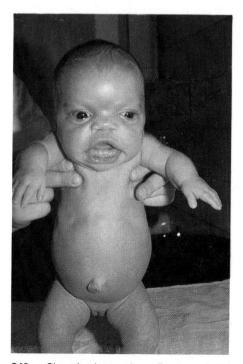

243 Chondrodystrophy. Four-week-old sister of the patient in Figs. 241 and 242. Note the Olympian forehead, retracted root of the nose, hypertelorism, big mouth, micromelia of the arms, frog belly.

Marfan's Syndrome

Definition

Marfan's syndrome (arachnodactyly) is an autosomal dominant, hereditary disease which is manifested by multiple aberrations of mesenchymal tissue derivatives.

Clinical Findings

Changes of the locomotor system, circulatory system, and the eyes dominate the multiform, variable symptomatology: abnormally long limbs, especially the distal extremities, funnel or pigeon chest, dolichocephaly, lax joints and ligaments, hypoplasia of muscles and fat, luxation of the lens with iridodonesis, degeneration of the aortic media and cardiac defects. Formes frustes may present an extremely asthenic habitus.

Treatment

There is no treatment.

Prognosis

Considering the great variety of combinations and manifestations, the prognosis for survival also varies. Because of increased susceptibility to pulmonary infections, severe forms of the disease will lead to early death.

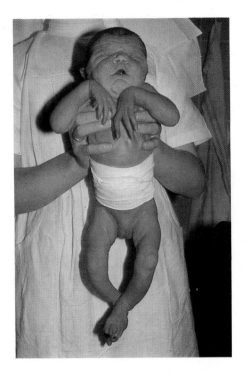

244   Marfan's syndrome in a newborn girl with unusually long hands and legs and "spider fingers." Hypoplasia of subcutaneous fatty tissue and muscles is evident.

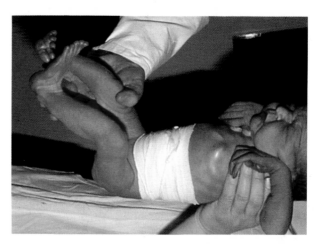

245 Abnormally long feet and hands. Loose skin. Slight generalized cyanosis owing to congenital heart disease.

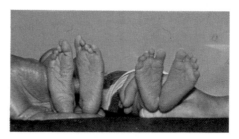

246 Arachnodactyly of feet compared to the normal feet of an infant of the same age.

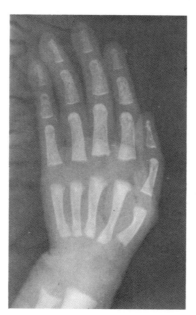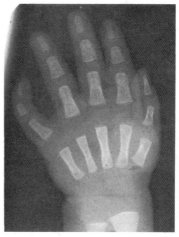

247 Radiogram of the hand compared to that of a normal child of the same age. Long hand, elongated diaphyses.

Maxillary Osteomyelitis

Definition

Maxillary osteomyelitis appears almost exclusively in infants during the first trimester. This hematogenous, severe form of osteomyelitis primarily affects dental germ.

Clinical Findings

Connected with pemphigoid, other staphylococcal infections, or even without recognizable primary bacterial focus, temperature will rise, and inflammatory swelling of cheek and eyelids appears on the affected side. A sanguinopurulent discharge appears at the palpebral fissure and nostril.

Sometimes the dental germ is expelled from the swollen alveolar process. Thrombosis of a sinus is a threatening complication.

Differential Diagnosis

A swollen and closed eye may be caused by maxillary osteomyelitis, orbital phlegmon, ethmoiditis, or sinus thrombosis.

Treatment

Immediate, massive administration of antibiotics may shorten or mitigate the process.

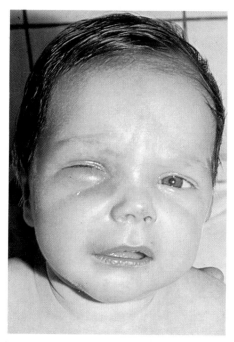

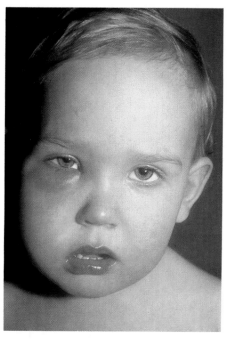

248   Right-sided maxillary osteomyelitis in a five-week-old infant. Postnatally, extensive pemphigoid, rise of temperature, vomiting, facial swelling, ESR 100/110. Sanguino-purulent nasal discharge containing staphylococcus aureus haemolyticus.

249   Right-sided ethmoid sinusitis following measles in a girl aged 22 months. High fever, ESR 55/100, leukocytes 17400/µl. On roentgenogram, ethmoid cells are opaque. Cured by erythromycin.

Parulis

Definition

In the presence of carious deciduous teeth with gangrenous pulp and apical parodontitis, recurrent submucous abscesses may arise at the gingival margin leading also to fistula formation. In case of recrudescence of this chronic apical parodontitis with more severe local and general signs of inflammation, a subperiosteal abscess of the jaw will follow; the disorder is called parulis.

Clinical Findings

At the alveolar gingival margin a red, granulomatous mucosal nodule appears. Its purulent content increases constantly until finally a fistula has been formed. Sudden onset of severe pains, collateral buccal edema, and elevated temperature are typical manifestations of parulis. A few days later the abscess perforates spontaneously into the oral cavity. Osteomyelitis of the jaw is a rare complication.

Treatment

Suppurative deciduous teeth ought to be extracted without concern for their function of preserving a particular space, because recurrent inflammations might damage the germ of the subsequent permanent tooth. Local treatment of acute parulis consists of intraoral incision, supported by antibiotic therapy.

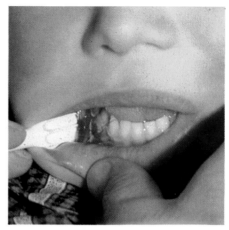

250   Submucosal alveolar abscess originating from the deciduous molar in the right lower jaw of a four-year-old boy. ESR 38/64. Extraction resulted in cure.

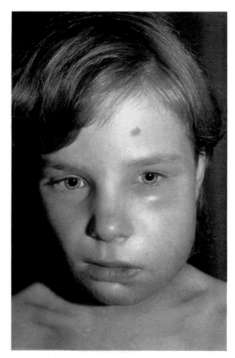

251   Parulis. The hard and extremely painful buccal swelling disappeared after spontaneous perforation of a subperiosteal abscess into the oral cavity. The abscess was situated alongside the third mandibular deciduous molar.

Funnel Chest

Definition

Pectus excavatum is a constitutional, often familial depression deformity of the anterior thoracic wall. The mesosternum is displaced dorsally.

Clinical Findings

The hollow excavation of the anterior thoracic wall shows paradoxal depression on inspiration. About two-thirds of the cases progress during growth, but narrowing of the intrathoracic space seldom causes organic complaints (increased rate of bronchopulmonary infections, cardiac arrhythmias).

Treatment

Arrest of funnel chest progression may be attempted by exercises, most of all by swimming. In severe cases surgery is indicated.

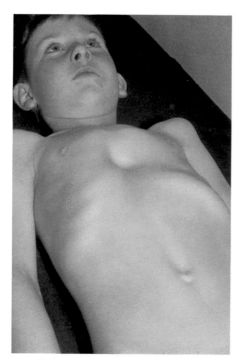

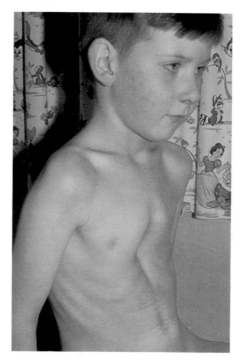

252   Funnel chest in a boy aged seven years. There were no organic complaints, but neurotic disturbances were reported.

253   Paradoxical respiration in this child: deepening of the excavation during inspiration. The thoracic spine is kyphotic.

Congenital Clubfoot

Definition

Pes equinovarus is a genetic, congenital deformity of the foot. Disturbance of muscular development is probably the primary cause of the disorder. The incidence is one to two per thousand newborns. It is twice as high in boys as in girls. In slightly more than half of the cases the malformation is bilateral. In 10 to 20 per cent there is a familial trait.

Clinical Findings

The three characteristic components of clubfoot deformity are explained by the Latin expression of *pes equinovarus adductus:* talipes equinus, supination and adduction of the anterior foot. Supination of the posterior part of the foot is the most detrimental factor: the calcaneus is elevated and displaced medially.

Treatment

The position of the foot is corrected manually on the first or second day of life. Overcorrection is fixed by a classical cast or Browne splint, modified by Grob. Treatment is continued over six months. If the calcaneus cannot be corrected, achillotomy must be done. The rate of recurrence is high in clubfoot. Even on immediate postnatal treatment it is almost 50 per cent.

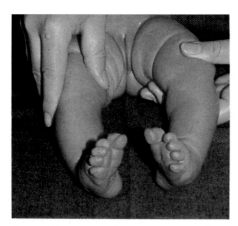

254   Bilateral clubfoot in a newborn girl. The characteristic calcaneal supination is well demonstrated.

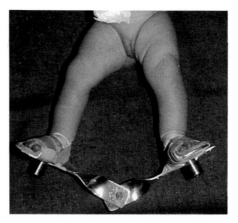

255   Reposition of clubfeet using Grob's modification of the Browne splint.

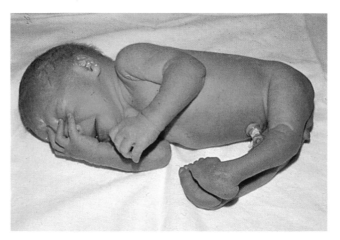

256   Marked neurogenic bilateral pes equinovarus in a newborn with lumbosacral meningomyelocele and paresis of the legs.

Congenital Dislocation of Hip

Definition

Congenital dislocation of the hip joint is probably caused by hereditary disturbances of estrogen catabolism (relaxin) in the mother, causing intrauterine weakening of the capsule of the joint. This facilitates dislocation of the femoral head with subsequent formation of osseous articular dysplasia. The incidence is 1 to 2 per 1000 and is five to six times higher in girls than in boys. In about 60 per cent of the cases the disorder is unilateral, in 40 per cent it is bilateral. Ten per cent of the affected children are delivered from breech presentation (compared to three to four per cent in the average population). In 20 per cent of the cases there is a familial trait.

Clinical Findings

Ortolani's phenomenon is the most important early sign during the neonatal period, indicating a tendency to luxation. Slow external rotation and abduction of the internally rotated leg with rectangular flexion of hip and knee causes distinct snapping of the femoral head. Later, abduction is limited, the gluteal fold lies high, and the leg is shortened. Trendelenburg's phenomenon can be demonstrated in the upright position: if weight is put on the luxated leg, the pelvis drops on the unaffected side. There is usually limping and waddling in the case of bilateral dislocation. Roentgenologic manifestations can also be demonstrated: steep cranial portion of the acetabulum with insufficient concavity, latero-cranial dislocation of femur, and interruption of Menard's line.

Treatment

The therapeutic principle consists of abduction of the reduced thigh in order to relieve the capsular tissue and to attain formative stimuli upon the acetabulum. In infancy, special diapers or Pavlik's bandage are useful. Overcorrected positions of the joint over long periods cause complicating necroses of the femoral head in 20 per cent of the cases (Perthes luxation).

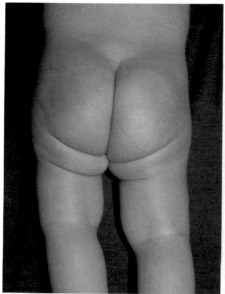

257 Left-sided congenital dislocation of the hip. The left gluteal fold is higher than the right. Ability to abduct is diminished.

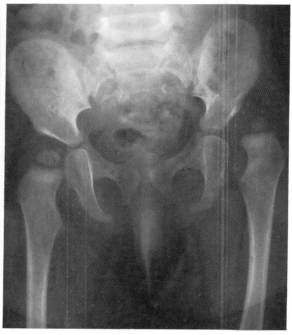

258 On the left: increased acetabular angle, displaced femoral head, and interrupted Menard's line. Ossification center of the left femoral head is smaller than the right.

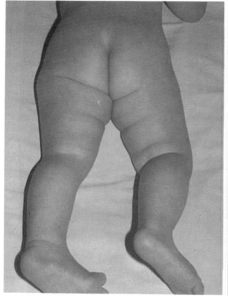

259 Incomplete dislocation of the left hip joint in a 20-month-old girl, who is not yet able to stand. Note the asymmetry of the gluteal folds. Congenital hip dislocation is also present in the infant's sister and maternal aunt.

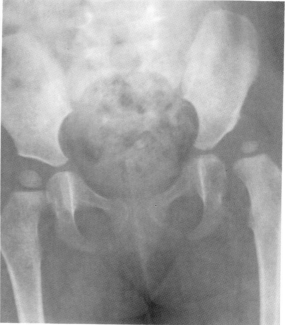

260 Increased acetabular angle on the left with the small femoral head dislocated latero-cranially; interrupted Menard's line.

Dermatoses

Congenital Ichthyosis

Definition

Congenital ichthyosis is an autosomal recessive hereditary disease. It is manifested by congenital anomalies of cornification of the skin. Depending on the severity of the disorder, a differentiation is made between grave congenital ichthyosis (fetal congenital ichthyosis, malignant keratoma) and mild congenital ichthyosis.

Clinical Findings

In grave congenital ichthyosis the babies are born wit parchment-cracked skin, containing deep fissures. It may resemble oil paper (collodion baby) and shows lamellar peeling. Ectropionized eyelids, fish mouth, deformed earlobes and plump extremities cause a bizarre appearance which is expressed by the term "harlequin fetus." In mild congenital ichthyosis, the same changes are present but are less severe.

Differential Diagnosis

In contrast to congenital ichthyosis, the more common disorder of ichthyosis vulgaris does not appear before the end of the first year. It does not affect bends of joints and axillary or gluteal folds and is preferably found on extensor sides of extremities. Hereditary transmission is autosomal dominant.

Treatment

Specific treatment does not exist. In the severe form, corticosteroids, ointments, and vitamin A are given. Infants affected by severe congenital ichthyosis die from infection within the first few weeks of life. Survival chances are good in mild forms of the disease.

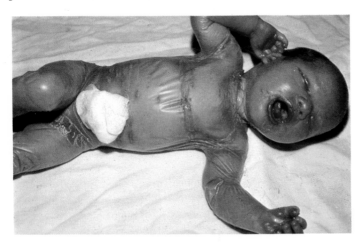

261 Ichthyosis congenita gravis in a newborn girl. Note the creased, cracked, parchmented skin in the joint bends.

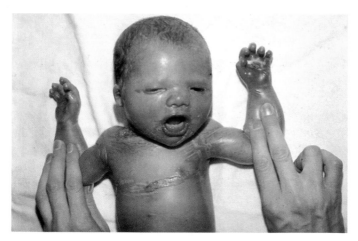

262   Bizarre features with ectropionated eyelids and "fish mouth." Onychogryposis of the fingernails.

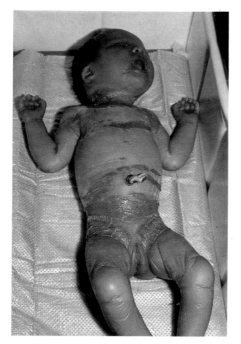

263   Second day of life. Large patches of abdominal skin begin to separate.

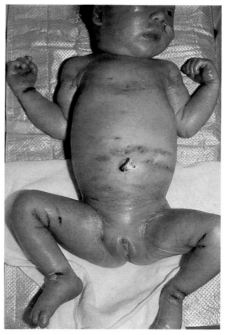

264   Eleventh day of life. Complete desquamation within ten days. Death from pneumonia on the 13th day of life. Seven of the same parents' 12 children are affected with congenital ichthyosis.

Epidermolysis Bullosa Hereditaria

Definition

Epidermolysis bullosa hereditaria is a hereditary dermatosis characterized by a tendency to vesiculation after minor mechanical irritation. Three different forms are defined depending on severity and hereditary transmission of the disease.

Clinical Findings

Epidermolysis bullosa hereditaria simplex is a dominant hereditary disease which appears in 50 per cent of the children of one affected parent. Generally it starts in the neonatal period and shows subcorneal vesicles. These appear on parts of the skin which are exposed to tangenital pressure. They heal without leaving scars. Nikolski's phenomenon is negative in most cases (separation of epidermis from corium after slight rubbing with fingernail). With growing age there is a certain tendency to regress. *Epidermolysis bullosa hereditaria dystrophica* is another dominant hereditary disease. Subepithelial vesicles arise also on portions of skin which are not exposed to pressure. Scars remain after healing. In most cases Nikolski's phenomenon is positive, nails are dystrophic and in about 20 per cent of the cases, mucous membranes are affected. The most serious form of the disease is called *Epidermolysis bullosa hereditaria dystrophica polydysplastica.* It is a recessive hereditary disorder and appears in 25 per cent of children of parents with normal phenotype and pathologic genotype. Even in the newborn, ubiquitous subepithelial vesicles are present on skin and mucous membranes. Healing proceeds with scarry atrophy. Nikolski's phenomenon is positive, dystrophies of nails and malformations of other organs may be found. Prognosis is doubtful.

Treatment

There is no special treatment. Therapeutic efforts concentrate on prevention of mechanical irritation and infection as well as application of corticosteroids and antibiotics.

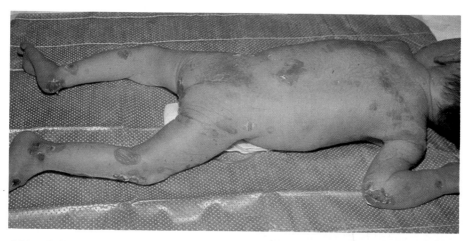

265 Epidermolysis bullosa hereditaria dystrophica, eighth day of life. Multiple vesicles already at birth. Positive Nikolski's sign. Double consanguinity of the grandparents.

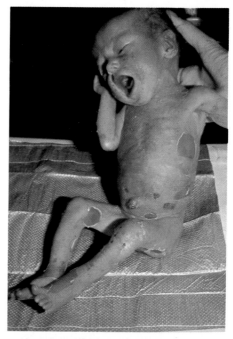

266 Nineteenth day of life. Increasing number of rapidly rupturing vesicles. Vesicular content sterile.

267 Twentieth day of life. Vesiculation also occurred on the hairy scalp and duodenal atresia was also present. Death at the age of three weeks.

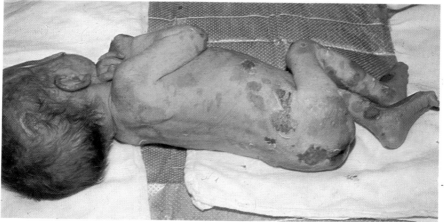

Pigmented Nevi

Definition

The clinical term pigmented nevus includes three forms of nevi with different histopathology (pigmented nevus or mole means a constitutional, circumscript, cutaneous malformation).

1. Accumulation of melanin in basal epidermal cells which are unable to produce their own pigment: ephelide, nevus spilus.
2. Increased number of pigment-forming melanocytes in the deeper corium: mongolian spot, blue nevus.
3. Increased number of modified melanocytes (nevus cells) on the border between epidermis and corium: nevus-cell nevus, juvenile melanoma (Spitz).

Clinical Findings

Nevus spilus is a light-brown hyperpigmentation (café-au-lait spot) of variable size and limits. It appears most commonly on the trunk. Larger numbers are present in neurofibromatosis (Recklinghausen's disease) and in Albright's syndrome. *Mongolian spot* is peculiar to the Mongol race. In one to three per cent this bluish spot appears also in European races. With growing thickness of the skin it disappears after a few years. *Blue nevi* are rare, flat or elevated solitary nodules with color varying from brown-black to blue, corresponding to the depth of melanocytes in the corium. *Nevus-cell nevus* is the most common pigmented nevus of childhood. It may be flat, elevated, verrucous or hairy and may, like fur, cover larger portions of the body (hairy nevus). Clinically nevus-cell nevus and *juvenile melanoma* cannot be differentiated. The latter appears between the third and thirteenth year of age and usually affects the face. Nevus-cell nevus and juvenile melanoma are potentially malignant disorders. On the other hand, they hardly ever undergo malignant degeneration during childhood, and in the adult very rarely, despite their high incidence (about one in one million).

Treatment

Solitary nevus-cell nevus and juvenile melanomas can be surgically removed. The previous fear that the manipulation provokes malignant degeneration is unfounded.

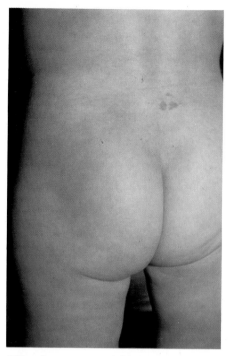

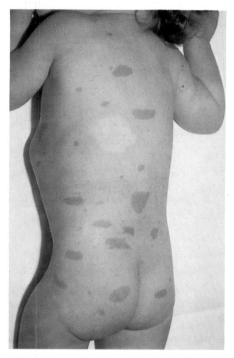

268 Large mongoloid spot on the left gluteal region. Age of the boy: 14 months.

269 Disseminated nevi spili (café-au-lait spots) and scattered depigmentations. Eight-month-old infant whose mother shows the same cutaneous changes.

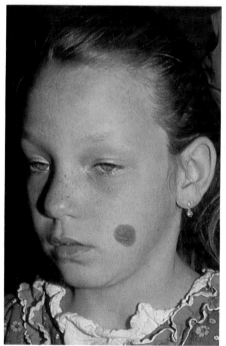

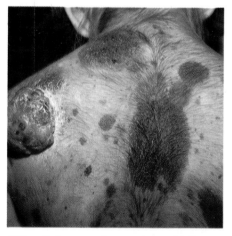

270 Slightly hairy nevus-cell on the cheek. Freckles on the bridge of the nose. Age of the girl: seven years.

271 Hairy nevus in a newborn girl. Deeper, partly hyperkeratotic nevi within the corium. A bluish hue and more superficial, reddish-brown borderline nevi can be seen.

Nevus Flammeus (PORT-WINE STAIN)

[handwritten:] same as vasular ectasia

Definition

Nevus flammeus (capillary hemangioma, port-wine mark) is a telangiectatic disorder with median or unilaterial localization. In the nuchal or frontal area of almost every second newborn a nevus flammeus is found. Lateral nevus flammeus is present in the trigeminal area in Sturge-Weber syndrome, and on the extremities in Klippel-Trenaunay syndrome.

level. Media nevi show a great tendency to regress. This is not the case with lateral, often segmentally distributed nevi. In Sturge-Weber syndrome there are unilateral facial nevi, intracranial calcifications, convulsions, and glaucoma caused by angiomatous changes of pia mater and the choroid membrane of the eye. Klippel-Trenaunay syndrome is characterized by hypertrophy of soft tissue and bones in the telangiectatic extremity.

Clinical Findings

Nevus flammeus, pale to flame red and sharply limited, lies within the cutaneous

Treatment

There is no treatment. *[handwritten:] cosmetic — argon laser*

[handwritten:] nevus flammeus of trigiminal area → component of s-w-syndrome.

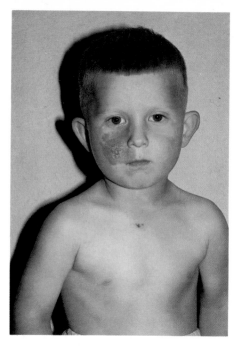

272 Lateral facial nevus in the area of the second trigeminal branch. Four-year-old boy without any further evidence of Sturge-Weber syndrome.

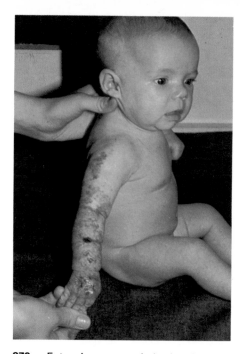

273 Extensive, congenital telangiectases and phlebectasias on the arm of a two-month-old infant. Ulcerations on lower arm and dorsum of hand.

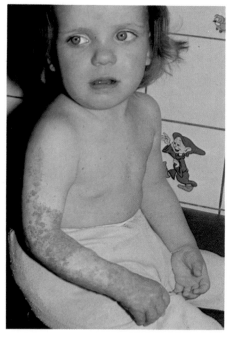

274 Infant in Fig. 273 at the age of two years: Partial involution of angiectases without any treatment.

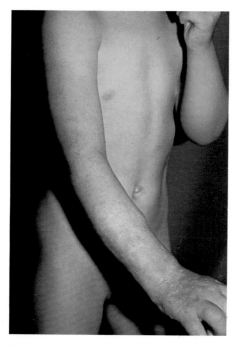

275 Almost complete spontaneous regression of the vascular nevus (child in Figs. 273 and 274 at the age of three and one-half years). Hypertrophy of the lower arm now becomes evident, as in Klippel-Treanaunay syndrome.

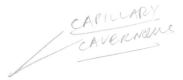

CAPILLARY
CAVERNOUS

Hemangioma

Definition

Hemangioma is a benign tumorous change of blood vessels. It appears chiefly in small infants, the incidence in girls is twice as high as in boys. In 20 per cent of the cases the disorder is disseminated.

Clinical Findings

Planotuberous hemangioma is slightly elevated, finely granulated, bright red and can be squeezed out. Tuberonodose hemangioma, which is found less frequently, is nodular, grossly granulated and of darker red color. Hemangioma lies subcutaneously and appears as a soft, cutaneous bulge that shines through the skin with a bluish-gray hue. Congenital giant hemangioma combined with thrombocytopenic purpura is called Kasabach-Merritt syndrome. Most hemangiomas arise during the first three months of life. From the sixth month of life until puberty more than 90 per cent have disappeared spontaneously, 70 per cent of them as early as infancy. Healing starts centrally despite primary peripheral enlargement.

Treatment

Cosmetically or functionally disturbing hemangiomas can be removed by surgical or radiologic intervention (soft rays, yttrium). Active treatment is a vital indication in Kasabach-Merritt syndrome. Because of the great tendency to spontaneous healing, it is worth while postponing treatment.

R c̄. steroids

- may consider s̄
excision in
cavernous hemangioma

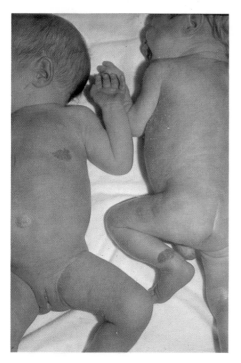

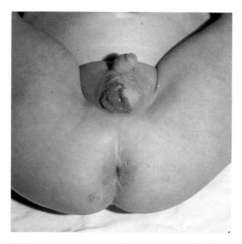

276   Typical planotuberous hemangiomas in newborn twins. Additional finding: two vaccination weals on the left thigh immediately after BCG vaccination.

277   Hemangioma of the scrotal skin in a one-year-old. Any trial of active treatment at this site would be malpractise.

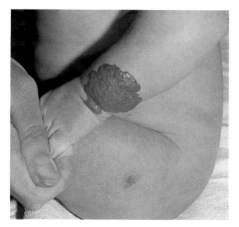

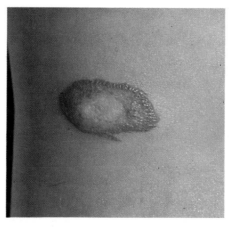

278   Planotuberous hemangioma on the left forearm of a two-month-old infant. Additional finding: BCG vaccination scar seven weeks after intracutaneous vaccination.

279   Typical example of spontaneous regression of a planotuberous hemangioma. Six-month-old infant.

Cystic Lymphangioma of the Neck (BENIGN)

Defintion

Cystic lymphangioma of the neck, also called hygroma colli cysticum, is a benign, multilocular mass on the lateral portion of the neck. It is filled with liquid and caused by tumorous growth of lymph vessels. The disorder may be congenital or develop during the first year of life.

Clinical Findings

The subcutaneous tumor may reach the size of a child's head, its consistency is soft and elastic. A bluish color shines through the skin and the tumorous mass may invade the floor of the mouth, tongue, and mediastinum. Often there is no sharp demarcation against the surrounding tissue.

Differential Diagnosis

Lateral cyst of the neck (branchial cyst) always lies ventral to the superior portion of the sternocleidomastoid muscle. It will not grow larger than about 5×3 cm and the consistency is firmer than in lymphangioma. Subcutaneous, cavernous hemangioma is softer and can be squeezed out; submental teratoma lies closer to the midline and is harder than lymphangioma.

Treatment

Surgical extirpation after the first six months of life. Lymphangiomas do not respond to radiotherapy.

Prognosis

Growing tendency is small but there is no tendency to spontaneous healing either. Relapse is common after incomplete extirpation.

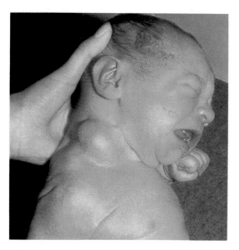

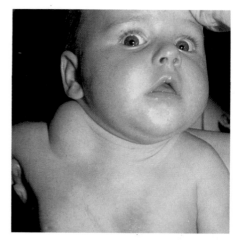

280   Plum-sized soft-elastic lymphangioma behind the sternocleidomastoid of a newborn. Note the bluish tinge in center of the tumor.

281   Cystic lymphangioma of the neck was already present at birth in this five-month-old girl.

Dermatitis Glutealis

Defintion

Perianal dermatitis is an inflammatory irritation of the skin in the genito-anal area of the newborn. Because of careless feeding it is caused by alkaline stools and urine (ammonia). Synonyms are: diaper dermatitis, dermatitis ammoniacalis, erythema gluteale papulosum, posterosivum or pseudosyphiliticum, dermatitis intertriginosa or simply intertrigo. The latter is a general expression for chafing in the area of skin folds (perianal, retroauricular, axillary) which may be caused by faulty care, ammonia or may be a manifestation of seborrheic dermatitis.

Clinical Findings

Redness, papules, pustules, erosions and, in serious cases, ulcerations, appear on genital organs, buttocks, and inner aspect of thighs. Development of gluteal dermatitis is favored by dyspepsia.

Differential Diagnosis

Candida-mycosis and early seborrheic dermatitis have to be excluded.

Treatment

Diapers should be changed frequently and the skin covered with cream or ointment; nonporous rubber pants should be avoided.

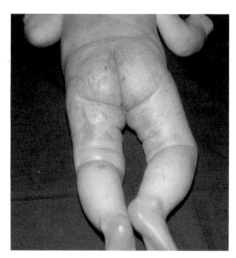

282 Gluteal dermatitis at the erythematous stage in a two-month-old infant. Dyspepsia.

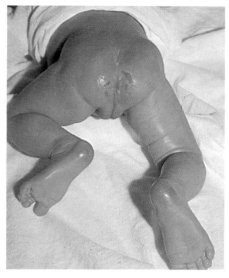

283 Gluteal dermatitis at the erosive stage in a five-week-old infant. Generalized cutaneous sensitivity, intertrigo of heels.

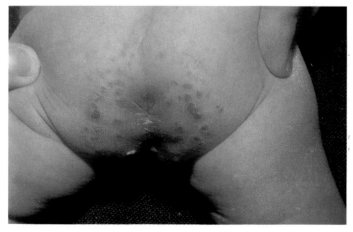

284 Post-erosive gluteal erythema in a neglected six-week-old infant.

Dermatitis Seborrhoides

Definition

Seborrheic dermatitis (eczema seborrhoicum) is a skin disease of the young infant, characterized by inflammatory erythrodermia with desquamation and seborrhea. The etiology is not known.

Clinical Findings

The basic efflorescence is a non-itching, fatty desquamative focus with a reddened base and a peripheral maximum of exudation. As early as the first trimester crusts on the scalp and intertrigo in the area of larger skin folds indicate the disease: behind ears, on neck, axillae, and in the area covered by diapers. Generally, healing occurs during the first year of life.

Differential Diagnosis

The disorder is differentiated from *endogenous eczema of the infant* by its early onset, lack of itching, increased incidence in nursing infants and better prognosis. Candida mycosis of the gluteal region (candidiasis glutealis, intertriginous candidiasis) with an enamel-like, shining red erythema and scaling border as well as localized distribution, may be mistaken for seborrheic dermatitis. Possible candida colpitis of the mother, oral candida infection of the infant, absence of the fatty component of desquamation, microscopic demonstration of monilia and good response to antimycotic drugs allow arrival at the right diagnosis.

Treatment

The principles of therapy consist of attentive care of the skin, local administration of mild ointments and prevention of infection.

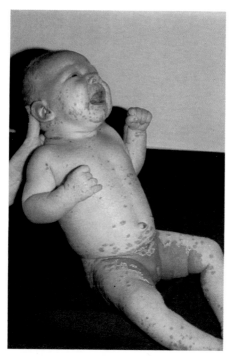

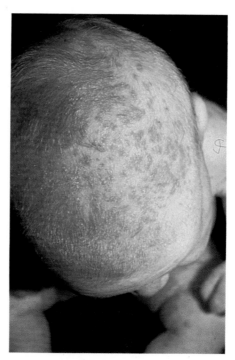

285 Seborrheic dermatitis in a six-week-old infant. Large erythematous patches are visible in the genitoanal region. Small spots are disseminated over the trunk and extremities.

286 Cradle cap in seborrheic dermatitis. Age of infant: five months.

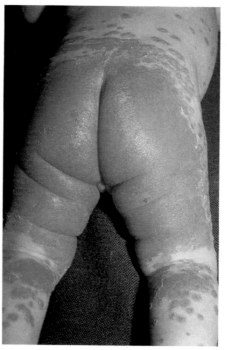

287 Typical flat erythema with scaling on its borders in the area covered by diapers.

Exfoliative Erythroderma (Leiner's Disease)

Definition

Today, Leiner's disease is a very rare disorder. It is the extreme variant of seborrheic dermatitis and primarily affects breast-fed infants during the first trimester.

Clincal Findings

Similar to seborrheic dermatitis, Leiner's disease starts with red, lamellar, desquamative spots on head and trunk. Predilected sites are the larger skin folds (neck, inguinal region). Later the disease rapidly spreads over the whole body. The fatty desquamation leaves bright-red, dry areas of skin. There is no itching. Complicating infections are common.

Treatment

Local treatment, prophylaxis against infections, and administration of corticosteroids are indicated.

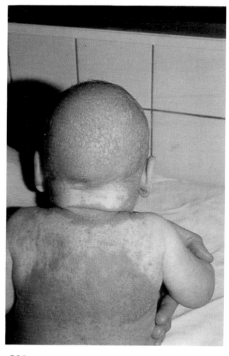

288

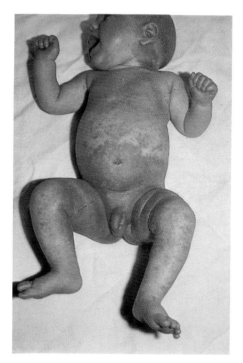

289

288–290 Generalized seborrheic, desquamative erythrodermia in a three-month-old, breast-fed infant. The changes have been present from the second month of life.

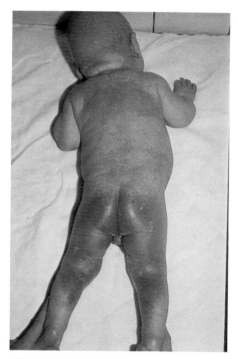

290

Endogenous Eczema

Definition

Endogenous eczema (atopic dermatitis, constitutional eczema, constitutional neurodermatitis) is the cutaneous form of reaction of genotypical-hereditary, atopic-allergic diathesis. Bronchial asthma and vasomotoric rhinitis are other manifestations of the same dysregulation. Morbidity is one to three per cent. Onset after the first trimester, a chronic intermittent course, deterioration in winter, and later simultaneous or alternating incidence of bronchial asthma are characteristic signs.

Clinical Findings

From the third month of life, atopic dermatitis is manifested by erythema, fine desquamation, formation of papules, vesicles, and crusts combined with oozing. Cheeks and scalp are predilected sites. During infancy and school age other signs predominate: disseminated, papular, single foci, as well as areas of lichenification on the trunk, extremities and flexor aspects of joints (neurodermatitis, Besnier's prurigo, lichen chronicus of Vidal, eczema of flexures). Severe itching with subsequent danger of impetigo is present during all stages.

Treatment

Combined therapy with administration of corticosteroids prefered.

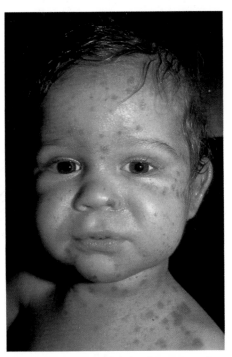

291   Constitutional infantile eczema in a 17-month-old boy. Itching, vesiculopapular, crusty efflorescences. Eosinophils at 12 per cent.

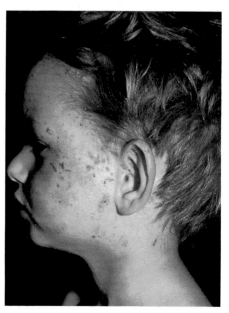

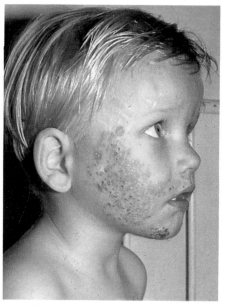

292 Endogenous eczema in a boy of three years, eleven months. Scratched, oozing, crusted, and impetiginized foci.

293 Endogenous eczema in a 19-month-old boy. Dry, severely itching, partly scratched efflorescences are evident in the face. The disorder commenced at the age of three months.

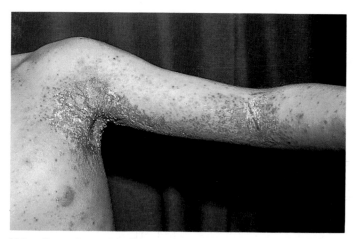

294 Neurodermatitis (flexural eczema) under corticoid treatment. Lichenified, shagreen, itching cutaneous changes in the folds of joint bends. Age of girl: 12 years.

Urticaria

Definition

Hives are an allergic skin disease. Development of edema in circumscript or larger skin areas accompanies acute appearance of multiple weals or angioneurotic edema (Quincke). Urticaria is not limited to any age group. The allergen is rarely found.

Clinical Findings

Urticarial eczema appears intermittently on trunk and extremities showing reddish or white, transient weals. These may rapidly change into convoluted or annular forms. Itching is always present, fever often so. Quincke's edema, covering larger areas, is mainly found on the face and neck, but also on hands and feet.

Treatment

Antipruritic agents, antihistamines, corticosteroids.

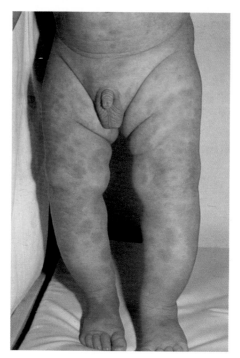

295 Generalized urticarial exanthem in an eight-month-old infant.

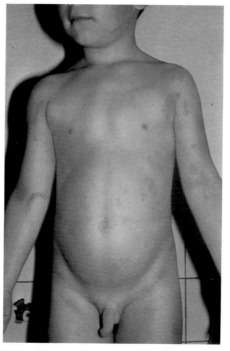

296 Discreet, but severely itching urticaria.. Quincke's edema of prepuce. Age of the boy: five years.

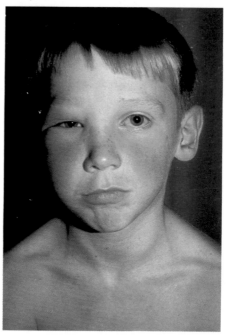

297 Quincke's edema of the right half of the face relapsing over four weeks; nine-year-old boy. One year previously Schönlein-Henoch purpura occurred; severe, hereditary allergy.

Impetigo Contagiosa

Definition

Impetigo contagiosa is a superficial pyodermia of high communicability. It appears most frequently in infants and is caused by streptococci, less commonly by staphylococci. Per contra, the skin of the newborn reacts to coccal infections with the formation of bullae.

Clinical Findings

Small vesicles, mainly on hairy scalp and face, rapidly change into characteristic yellow crusts which form on a red base. These may undergo polycyclic, convoluted, or disseminated expansion. With adequate treatment, impetigo will heal without leaving scars, having gone through a stage of red patches. Impetiginous nephritis is a rare complication.

Treatment

External application of antibiotics and prevention of autoinoculation by scratching.

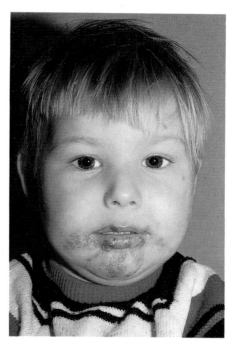

298   Impetigo contagiosa spreading to the labial mucosa (cheilitis impetiginosa). Age of the boy: three years.

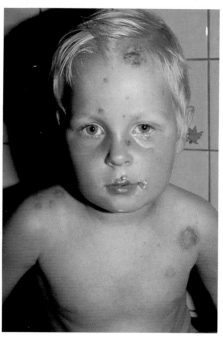

299   Disseminated impetiginous lesions in a boy of four years, six months.

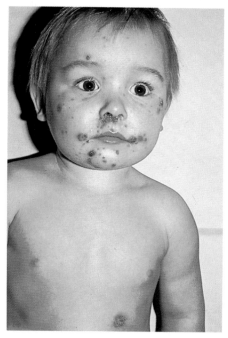

300   Staphylococcal impetigo contagiosa in a 30-month-old girl after severe pneumonia.

Tinea Inguinalis

Definition

Tinea inguinalis (jock itch, eczema marginatum) is a fungal skin disease, caused by epidermophyton floccosum or trichophyton mentagrophytes or rubrum. It is localized on the inner sides of the thighs. Contrary to the adult, it is a rare disease in infants just as vesicular, intertriginous or squamous-hyperkeratotic fungus infections of the hands and feet are rare in children.

Clinical Findings

Plaques are reddish-brown, round or polycyclic, and sharply circumscribed. Little desquamation at the slightly elevated border, itching is rare, and oozing is never found.

Differential Diagnosis

Differential diagnosis from seborrheic eczema (pityriasis marginata), erythema migrans originating from a tick bite, and erythema annulare centrifugum Darier (erythema gyratum perstans) may be difficult.

Treatment

Antimycotic agents are applied locally and griseofulvin internally. The tendency to relapse, however, is high.

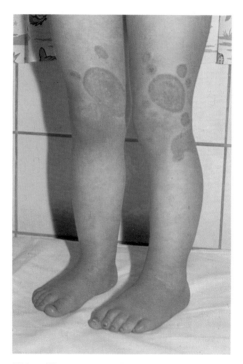

301 Tinea cruris. Typical discreet, peripheral scaling with a slightly elevated border. Two-year-old girl.

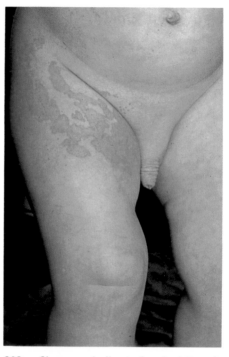

302 Changes similar to inguinal tinea in a one-year-old infant. No fungi demonstrated; histologically: vascular nevus.

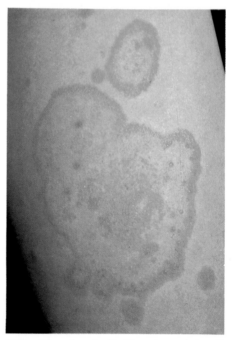

303 Tinea inguinalis. Note the peripherally small-vesicular lesions with brownish, central pigment, and polycyclic borders. Ten-year-old boy.

Scabies

Definition

Scabies is caused by *Sarcoptes scabiei.* It is a parasitic skin disease, which, under poor sanitary conditions, is transmitted from man to man. After an incubation period of three to six weeks the mite burrows several millimeters' length into the stratum corneum, forming a tunnel parallel to the surface.

Clinical Findings

The course of the burrows is short, linear or tortuous – the color in the beginning white, later turning darker to black. Hands, feet, genital area, axillary, and periumbilical regions are predilected sites. The face is never affected. A papulovesicular exanthem is a common concomitant finding. Unbearable itching, especially when warm at night leads to various scarifications and subsequent impetigo. Thus, the real disease is often concealed. Microscopic demonstration of mites or eggs confirms the diagnosis. Mites are removed from the deep end of a burrow with a pin.

Treatment

Gamma benzene hexachloride is the most effective scabicide.

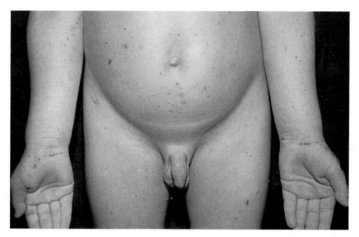

304 Scabies in a four-year-old boy from poor sanitary conditions. Numerous, mostly scratched, papules and burrows are evident. Note the cumulation over hand joints and abdomen.

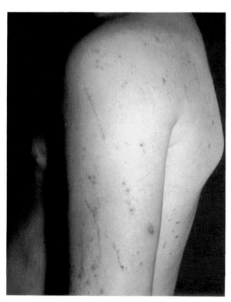

305 Burrows on the upper arm.

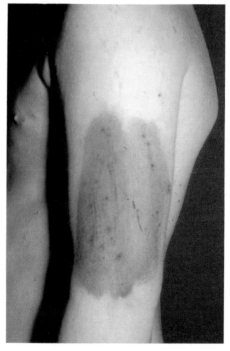

306 Burrows are better recognized by painting with ink.

Erythema Multiforme Exudativum

Definition

Erythema multiforme is an idiopathic, but in most cases a toxic-allergic skin disease characterized by polymorphous eruptions. Severe forms with increased involvement of mucous membranes (erythema exudativum multiforme majus) are also known as the Stevens-Johnson, Fiessinger-Rendu (Verosive pluriorificial ectodermosis), Baader and Fuchs syndromes.

Clinical Findings

Red spots of various sizes appear acutely, intermittently, and accompanied by elevated temperature. Any area of the body may be affected but extensor sides of extremities are predilected. The spots may become polycyclic or change into concentric rings. Vesiculopapular, urticarial, bullous, and hemorrhagic efflorescences may also be found. In erythema multiforme majus, erosive manifestations on mucous membranes and borderlines between skin and mucous membranes predominate (eyelids, lips, anus, genital organs). When without complications, the course of the disease is benign and will last from one to three weeks. But there is risk of relapse.

Treatment

Symptomatic.

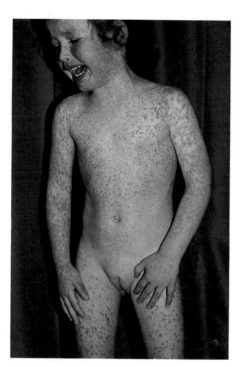

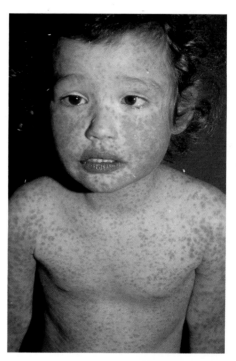

307   Erythema multiforme exudativum in a four-year-old girl; ninth day of penicillin treatment. Coarse, partly confluent (right lower arm), partly urticarial (thigh) exanthem. Septic temperature.

308   Isolated eruptions over upper right arm and left shoulder, showing concentric rings. Simultaneous affection of labial mucosa. Spontaneous healing after three weeks.

Psoriasis Vulgaris

Definition

Psoriasis is a hereditary parakeratosis with a chronic recurrent course. The low morbidity of about one per thousand indicates that during childhood it is a rare disorder compared to a tenfold frequency in the adult.

Clinical Findings

The individual psoriatic efflorescence has a red base covered with white scales. After slight touching, the fine, lamellar scales become more dictinct (candle-stain phenomenon). Fine hemorrhagic spots appear within the red base of the eruptions after removal of scales (dewdrop sign, Auspitz). Typical erythematous scaly patches may be found on the whole body including hairy portions of the head. Several forms are differentiated depending on the configuration of the lesions: psoriasis punctata, guttata, nummularis, or geographica. Itching is mainly present in repeat episodes.

Differential Diagnosis

Differential diagnosis can be difficult in certain forms of seborrheic eczema and tinea.

Treatment

Corticosteroids and antimetabolites may cause remissions.

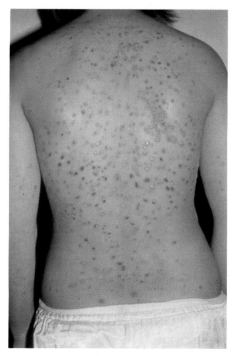

309 Psoriasis guttata, present for four weeks, caused severe scaling and itching. Age of the girl: 11 years.

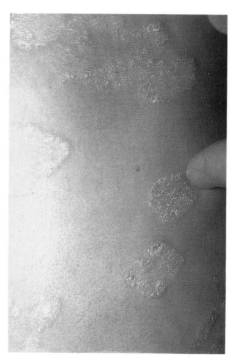

310 Acute attack of psoriasis nummularis in an eleven-year-old girl, who has been affected by the disorder for five years.

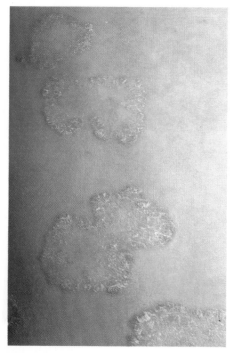

311 Gyrated and annular, separate psoriatic efflorescences.

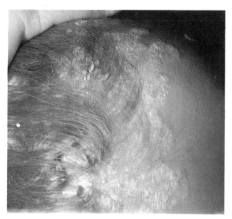

312 Extreme desquamation on the hairy skull.

Dermatitis Herpetiformis Duhring

Definition

Duhring's herpetiform dermatitis is a bullous dermatitis with a chronic intermittent course and unknown etiology.

Clinical Findings

Blisters occur on the whole body in groups resembling herpes but basically the skin remains unchanged, and the general state of health is hardly affected. In the adult, the polymorphous form predominates (vesicles, bullae, erythema, weals, pruritic eruptions) with concomitant itching and burning sensations. During childhood the monomorphous-bullous form without unpleasant sensations is more common. Face and mucous membranes are rarely affected. Nikolski's sign is negative. The vesicles contain eosinophils and the blood will often reveal eosinophilia.

Differential Diagnosis

The following vesiculo-bullous dermatoses must be excluded:
1. Pemphigus vulgaris, which is extremely rare during childhood. Only histologic examination will allow certain differentiation: intraepidermal vesiculation with akantholytic epithelial cells in pemphigus, corial vesicles without akantholysis in herpetiform dermatitis.
2. As genetic dermatosis, epidermolysis bullosa hereditaria (See p. 192).
3. As allergic dermatoses, vesiculo-bullous drug eruptions (See p. 192).

Treatment

No specific therapy. Prevention of infection. Symptomatic administration of corticosteroids.

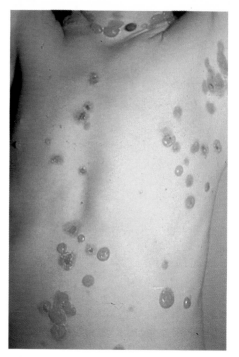

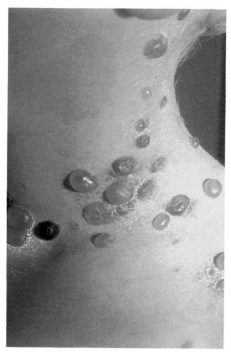

313 Dermatitis herpetiformis in a four-year-old boy (histologically confirmed). Painless eruption of smaller and larger vesicles started one week previously. The face and mucous membranes were not affected.

314 Groups of lentil to bean-sized, cutaneous efflorescences on the neck. Firm-elastic, drying, and hemorrhagic vesicles.

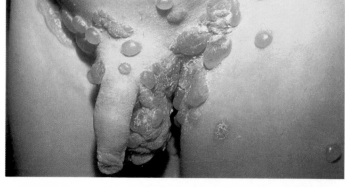

315 Primary efflorescences appear on the skin which shows no signs of any irritation. Vesicular content is clear and sterile in the beginning.

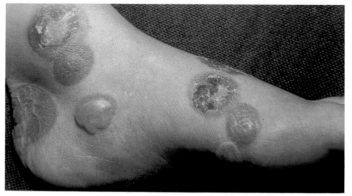

316 Primary and secondary efflorescences (vesicles, pustules, crusts) after four weeks of illness.

Disorders of the Nervous System

Spina Bifida

Definition

Idioplasmatic or exogenous inhibition of formation of the neural canal during the third week of embryonic life causes dorsal cleft formation of the spine (spina bifida). Meninges (meningocele) and cord (meningomyelocele) may present different extents of prolapse. The disorder appears two to three times per one thousand deliveries (stillbirths included); girls are twice as often affected as boys. Five to eight per cent of the siblings of these children show severe malformations of the central nervous system.

Clinical Findings

The lumbosacral region is the site of predilection for dysrhaphias. The least severe disorder is *spina bifida occulta.* It is characterized by cleft formation of vertebral arches. Retracted skin, hypertrichosis, nevus flammeus, or lipoma may be external manifestations of the disorder. In *meningocele,* a meningeal sac filled with spinal fluid protrudes through the separated vertebral arches (spina bifida cystica). Nervous elements are not affected and neurologic disturbances are missing. Pressure on the cyst causes tension of the anterior fontanel and diaphanoscopy reveals homogeneous transillumination. *Mengingomyelocele* is characterized by additional fissuration and prolapse of the cord. It is open either as a central dark-red medullovascular zone surrounded by a greyish-blue, so-called epithelioserosal zone, or it may be covered by a thin epithelial layer. Neurologic disturbances are present: flaccid paresis of legs with clubfoot, cystoplegia, and proctoplegia. Hydrocephalus, cranial defects, and the Arnold-Chiari syndrome are often found simultaneously. Ascending infections of meninges and urinary tract are threatening complications.

Treatment

Early surgical intervention.

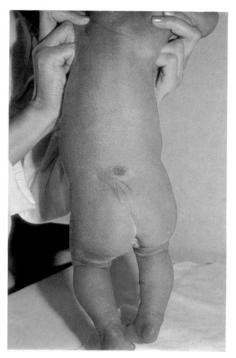

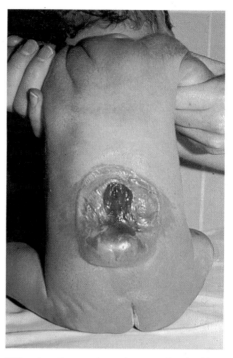

317 Spina bifida occulta with thinned skin and hypertrichosis. No neurologic deficiencies. Vertebral arches S_1 and S_2 appear open on roentgenograms.

318 Lumbosacral meningomyelocele. Note the central opening of the neural plate (medullovascular zone), and in the periphery, greyish-blue, shiny pia mater (epithelioserosal zone). Paresis of the legs is also evident.

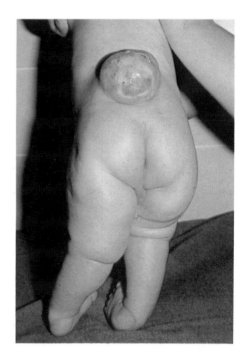

319 Epithelialized lumbosacral meningomyelocele in a three-month-old twin. Paralyses of the legs, bilateral neurogenic clubfeet, and permanent dripping of urine are evident. Among nine siblings there is another case of meningomyelocele.

Cranial Dysrhaphia

Definition

Cleavage in the area of the cranium is caused by inhibition of formation of the cranial neural canal. There may be various grades of inhibition. Similar to disturbances of junction of the spinal cord, cleavage is determined during the third week of embryonic life. The incidence in girls is two to three times higher than in boys. Familial traits occur.

Clinical Findings

The most common disorder of the kind is occipital cleavage with *meningocele* or *occipital encephalo-meningocele*. In *hemicephaly*, only parts of occipital and temporal bones remain as remnants of the bony cranial convexity (hemicrania). A dark red convolution of cerebral and meningeal rudiments presents on the base of the skull. *Anencephaly* is the highest grade of the disorder. Bony cranium and brains are completely absent. The infants are not viable.

Treatment

Cranial meningocele can be corrected by neurosurgical measures. Surgery should be performed during the first four weeks of life.

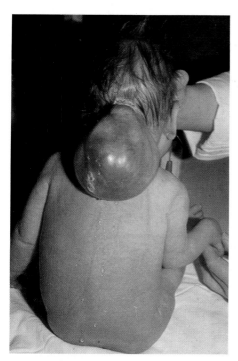

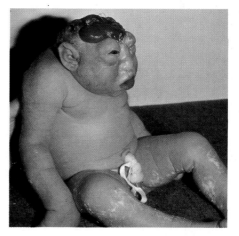

320   Occipital meningocele; CSF dripping from two spontaneously perforated orifices. Death occurred from meningitis after two months.

321   Hemicephaly. Frog-like features owing to prominent orbital cavities and short neck. Central respiratory disturbance.

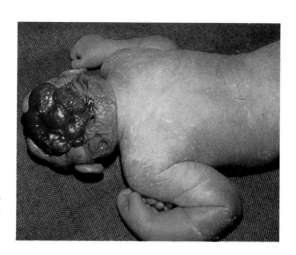

322   Occipital bone, temporal bone, and nondifferentiable cerebral remnants are present. Death occurred on the fourth day of life.

Moebius' Nuclear Aplasia

Definition

Moebius' syndrome is a congenital paretic disorder caused by primary aplasia of cerebral nerve nuclei. Paretic manifestations may be singular or multiple. They may be combined with malformations of the external and internal ear, micrognathia, and hypertelorism. In 30 per cent of the cases the disease is familial.

Clinical Findings

The most common pareses are the following:
1. *Congenital ptosis:* paralysis of levator palpebrae superioris muscle or the oculomotor nerve, with or without disturbance of bulbus-motility (temporal deviation of the eyeball).
2. *Congenital paresis of the abducens nerve:* There is internal rotation of the eyeball and enophthalmos.
3. *Congenital facial palsy:* especially of the inferior branch (paralysis of lips). Combination with other defects is common.

Differential Diagnosis

For the diagnosis of congenital facial palsy, birth trauma must be excluded.

Treatment

Ptosis and abducens paresis can be corrected by surgery.

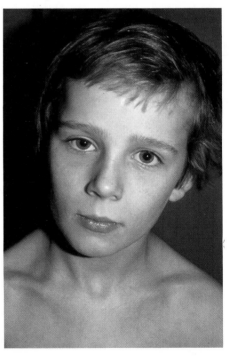

323   Discreet manifestation of congenital, right-sided ptosis (paresis of oculomotor nerve) with compensatory inclination of the head to the left. Simultaneous legasthenia occurred.

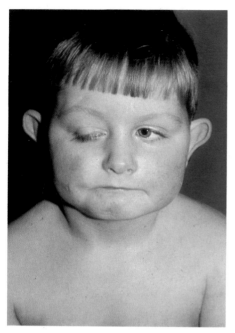

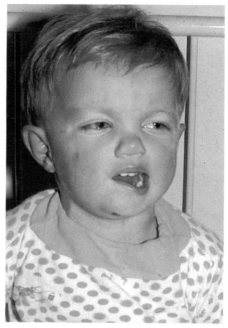

324   Congenital ptosis of the right side. Age of the boy, five and one-half years. Spoon-shaped ears.

325   Congenital paresis of the right lower branch of the facial nerve. Right earlobe poorly molded. No other defects.

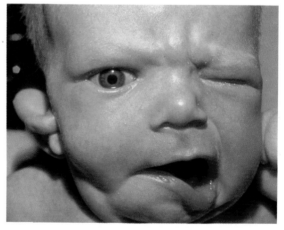

326   Right-sided congenital facial palsy affecting all three branches. No traumatic birth. Malformation of right external ear; age of the infant, four weeks.

Melkerssohn-Rosenthal Syndrome

Definition

Chronic relapsing facial swelling of unknown origin, associated with facial palsy has been named Melkerssohn-Rosenthal syndrome. The monosymptomatic form of the disease, which only shows swelling of lips, is called Miescher's syndrome.

Clinical Findings

The triad of labial swelling (granulomatous cheilitis, tapir mouth), peripheral facial palsy (33 per cent of the cases), and scrotal tongue (20 per cent of the cases) is completed by facultative appearance of epiphora ("crocodile tears" syndrome), salivation, swelling of regional lymph nodes, and dementia.

Differential Diagnosis

Quicke's edema, inflammatory edema of lips, rheumatic facial palsy.

Treatment

There is no treatment.

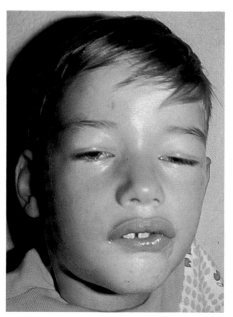

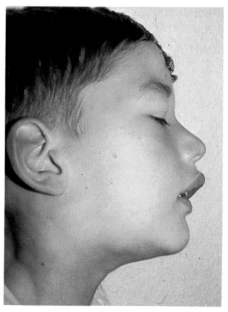

327 Facies in Melkerssohn-Rosenthal syndrome. Discreet facial palsy on the right, and lymphoma of the right neck are evident. Seven-year-old with convulsive disease.

328 Tapir mouth in Melkerssohn-Rosenthal syndrome.

Meningococcal Meningitis

Definition

Meningitis epidemica is caused by *Neisseria meningitidis* (Gram-negative diplococci). Meningococcal septicemia follows hematogenous spread of the infective organisms into the meninges. Communicability is low and in contrast to its name, epidemic appearance seldom occurs.

Clinical Findings

In the older infant several findings are typical for the disease: acute onset with headaches, fever, vomitting, nuchal rigidity and stupor, herpes labialis and embolic cutaneous hemorrhages the size of a few millimeters to about one centimeter. Serious forms are characterized by opisthotonos, convulsions, and loss of consciousness. During infancy, symptomatology is less complete. Tense or bulging fontanel is an important diagnostic criterion. Diagnosis is confirmed by pleocytosis exceeding 15,000 white cells, as well as demonstration of the organisms in the cerebrospinal fluid.

Treatment

Lethality has been lowered to five per cent since the introduction of chemotherapy; residual neurologic defects decreased to 10 to 20 per cent. Formerly, sulfonamides were used, today high doses of penicillin are administered.

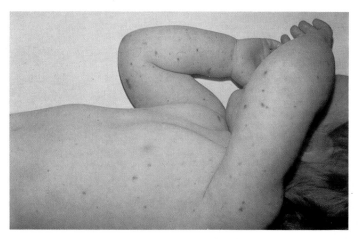

329 Cutaneous hemorrhage in a two-year-old girl with meningo-coccal meningitis. Vomiting, somnolence, no fever, purulent CSF, 42,000 cells per μl.

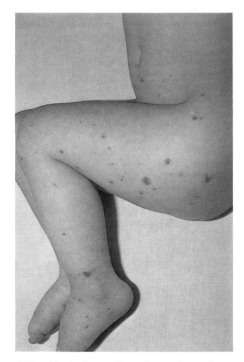

330 Typical manifestations of meningo-coccal purpura: large, dark-blue hemor-rhages with crenated borders (cutaneous embolism) and fleabite petechiae (toxic capillary damage). Sporadic, pinhead-sized, pale-red spots (allergic exanthem).

Waterhouse-Friderichsen Syndrome

Definition

The fulminant form of meningococcal sepsis is called Waterhouse-Friderichsen syndrome. Shock and hemorrhagic signs which are caused by endotoxins correspond to the Shwartzman-Sanarelli phenomenon with microthromboses and intravascular clotting. Peracute septicemia appears in about one per cent of manifest meningococcal infections.

areas (intravital livor mortis) are clinical signs of severe shock. Within a few hours numerous hemorrhagic spots appear in the skin, their size varying from a few millimeters to about one centimeter. The patient dies within eight to twenty-four hours, before meningitic changes are evident in the cerebrospinal fluid. Meningococci can be cultured from blood and cerebrospinal fluid. At autopsy hemorrhages can be found in all internal organs, including adrenals.

Clinical Findings

Acute onset of fever, vomiting, loss of consciousness, pallor (circulatory centralization), and livid spots on dependent body

Treatment

Rapid stabilization of circulatory system, and administration of penicillin and heparin is a favored course.

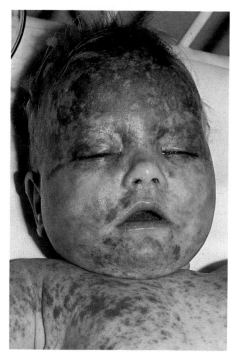

331 Waterhouse-Friderichsen syndrome in an eight-month-old girl. Deep uncons-ciousness, temperature 40.5°C, multiple, partly confluent cutaneous hemorrhages, bloody tears and saliva.

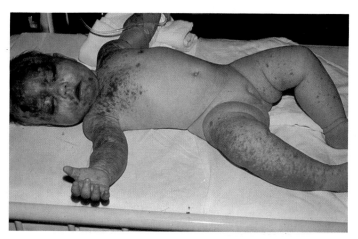

332 Intravital livor mortis on the lateral side of the right lower leg. Death within 18 hours after commencement of the disease.

Encephalitis

Definition

Most cerebral inflammations of childhood are caused by viruses; either primarily, as for instance by coxsackie, ECHO, arbo, herpes, or rabies viruses, or secondarily by postinfectious, neuro-allergic processes following measles, chickenpox, mumps, rubella, infectious mononucleosis, or vaccination against smallpox or rabies.

Clinical Findings

Manifestations of central irritations in acute encephalitis are extremely variable. Disturbances of consciousness, manifestations of hyperactivity or paralysis, hyperpyrexia, "cri encéphalique," and salivation are essential findings in the *encephalitic syndrome*. In cerebrospinal fluid protein and the number of cells are slightly elevated; glucose is distinctly elevated. In meningeal involvement, additional signs of the *meningitic syndrome* are found. The latter is characterized rather by signs of raised cerebral pressure (vomiting, bradycardia, headache, tense fontanel), and meningeal irritation.

Treatment

Since there is no treatment for viral encephalitis, persistent postencephalitic brain damage is common. It is manifested by signs of neurologic and mental deficiency syndromes.

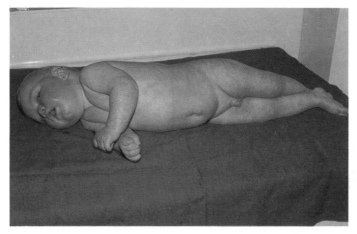

333   Encephalitis caused by herpes virus in a seven-month-old infant. Unconsciousness, alternating atony, hypertonic movement and tonic-clonic convulsions occurred owing to opisthotonos.

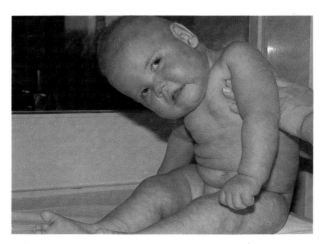

334   Atony, bulbar deviation. Residual syndrome of severe neurologic and mental deficiency.

Hydrocephalus

Definition

Enlargement of CSF spaces, called hydro-cephalus, may be caused by different disturbances: blocked passage of CSF (occlusive hydrocephalus), disturbed absorption of CSF (aresorptive hydrocephalus), increased production of CSF (hypersecretory hydrocephalus); or secondarily, by atrophy of cerebral mass (hydrocephalus e vacuo, passive or concomitant hydrocephalus). The great majority of the cases consists of occlusive and aresorptive forms. They are caused by malformation, inflammation, or hemorrhage causing occlusions in the area of the aqueduct and foramina Magendie and Luschka. The incidence of conatal hydrocephalus is one in 500 to 1500 deliveries.

Clinical Findings

In the newborn, elevated intracranial pressure causes enlargement of the skull with separation of sutures dehiscence and bulging of fontanels, prominence of cranial veins, and caudal and lateral displacement of the eyeballs (sunset look). In older children with synostosed cranial sutures, elevated cerebral pressure is manifested by headache, vomiting, choked disc, and optic atrophy. In cerebral atrophy, above all, the subarachnoidal space is enlarged (external hydrocephalus). In this case, pressure is not elevated and cranial circumference not increased. Microcephaly is more likely to appear.

Treatment

Operative treatment consists of CSF drainage from the lateral ventricle through a ventriculo-auricular shunt from the jugular vein into the right atrium (valvular drainage of Spitz-Holter or Pudenz-Heyer).

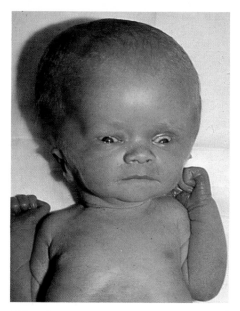

335 Congenital hydrocephalus of unknown etiology in a newborn. Head circumference 52 cm (normally 34 cm). "Sunset phenomenon."

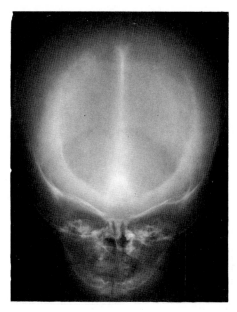

336 Pneumencephalogram at the age of four weeks. Marked symmetrical enlargement of lateral ventricles.

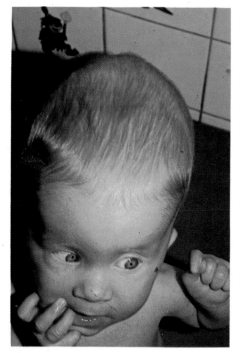

337 At the age of four months, two months after a Pudenz-Heyer operation, regression of head circumference from 61 cm before surgery to 53 cm. Behavior corresponds to age.

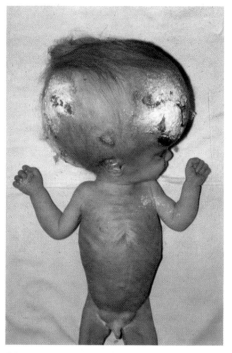

338 Excessive hydrocephalus of unknown origin in a 15-month-old twin. Decubitus ulcers.

Spastic Hemiplegia

Definition

Infantile spastic hemiplegia is a variant of infantile cerebral paresis. Similar to other forms (tetraplegia, paraplegia, athetosis, and atonic-astatic syndrome), it may be the result of prenatal, perinatal, or postnatal cerebral lesions caused by hypoxemic, hemorrhagic, or inflammatory disorders. After postnatal brain damage (e. g., encephalitis), spastic hemiplegia is more common than other forms.

Clinical Findings

Lowered activity of one arm or increased fist-making with inverted thumbs are among the first signs. They are followed by spastic hypertonia with exaggerated reflexes and pyramidal signs, and finally by flexion-contractures and foot drop. Generally, the upper extremity is more affected than the lower one. Frequent associated signs are: strabismus, disordered hearing and speech, hemiatrophy, convulsions, and dementia.

Treatment

Early special physiotherapy is the most important measure.

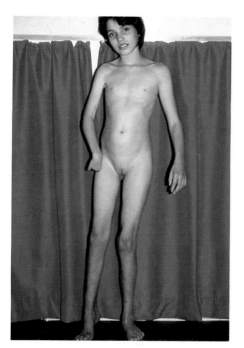

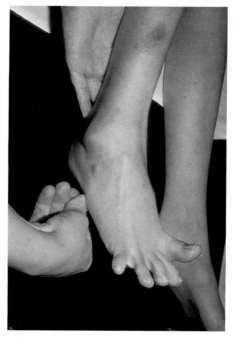

339   Twelve-year-old girl with right-sided spastic hemiplegia after measles ence-phalitis at the age of two years. Hemiatrophy, talipes equinus and typical inclination of the head toward the affected side are evident. Concomitant diabetes mellitus.

340   Babinski's sign.

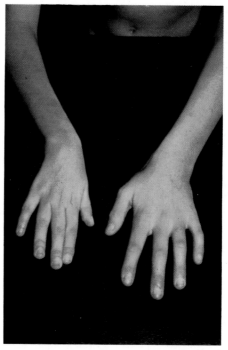

341   Marked atrophy of the spastic hand.

Tuberous Cerebral Sclerosis   (Auto. Dom.)

Definition

Tuberous sclerosis (Bourneville's disease) is a dominant hereditary disease belonging to the group of phacomatoses. They are characterized by multilocular tumorous formations according to the disturbed differentiation of tissue in early embryonic life (dysontogenetic process with blastomatous tendency). In Bourneville's disease tumors are found in brain (glycogen-containing proliferations of glia), retina, skin, heart, and kidneys.

Clinical Findings

Several disorders may be present in different combinations and grades: epilepsy, oligophrenia, cerebral disturbances of motion, and cutaneous changes such as multiple yellowish-red papules in the face (adenoma sebaceum, Pringle's nevus), gingival overgrowth, periungual fibroma (Koenen's tumors) and lumbosacral elastoma or connective tissue nevi (shagreen skin). Circumscript depigmentation may be an early cutaneous sign. On roentgenograms, calcified intracranial gliomas may be demonstrable.

Differential Diagnosis

In abortive forms with dermatologic signs as the only manifestation of the disease, it may be difficult to exclude von Recklinghausen's neurofibromatosis. Tumors of peripheral nerves never appear in tuberous sclerosis.

Treatment

There is no treatment. Anticonvulsive drugs must be given for epilepsy.

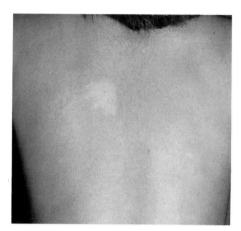

342   Foci of depigmentation in tuberous sclerosis. Four-year-old debilitated girl with nodding spasms.

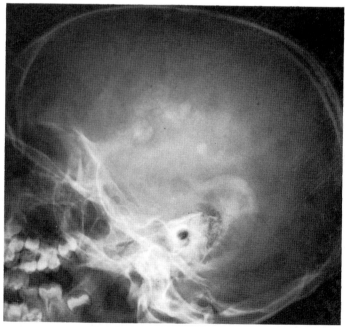

343   Disseminated intracranial calcifications over the middle cranial fossa.

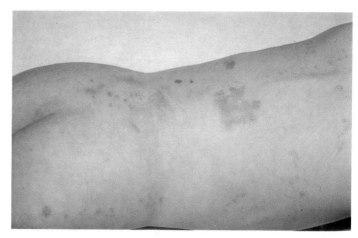

344 Lawn-like lumbosacral proliferations of connective tissue (elastic nevus) in tuberous sclerosis. Nine-year-old boy with convulsive disease and debility. Another case of epilepsy is present among his five siblings. The mother is affected by Pringle's syndrome.

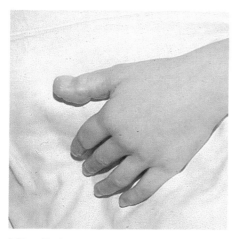

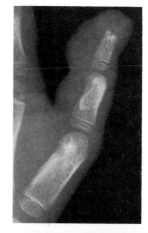

346

345 Periungual fibromas of the thumb.

346 Tuberous sclerosis. Destructive osseous processes in the distal phalanx of the thumb located at the homogeneous thickening of the cortical layer of the first-metacarpal.

347 Adenoma sebaceum on wing of the nose and neck. Mother of the child in Figs. 344 to 346.

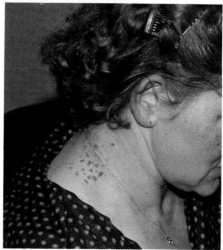

347

Neurofibromatosis   (AUTOS. DOMINANT)

Definition

Von Recklinghausen's neurofibromatosis is a dominant-hereditary, dysontogenetic disorder with a blastomatous tendency (phacomatosis). The disease originates in the nervous system and is charcterized by generalized perineural, cutaneous fibromas, neurinomas of the peripheral and central nervous system, and pigmented cutaneous spots.

Clinical Findings

The symptoms of the disease develop slowly. In early childhood there are usually only light-brown, pigmented spots (café-au-lait spots). Later, disseminated, soft, subcutaneous, and intracutaneous neurofibromas appear. They disappear on pressure and rebound with ceasing pressure. Moreover, on extremities, tumors form along the trunks of nerves. They are painful on pressure. Intraspinal and intracranial tumors may also appear, accompanied by corresponding neurologic symptoms. Circumscript giant-growth may occur.

Treatment

There is no treatment.

MANIFESTATIONS

- neurofibromas
- cafe-au-lait
- shagreen patch
- mental def.
- adenoma sebaceum
- seizures
- intracranial calcif'
- pheochromocytoma
- bone lesions
- phacomatosis

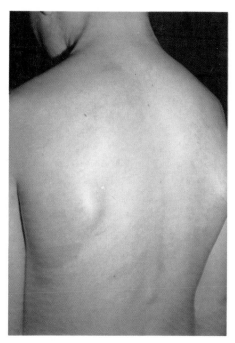

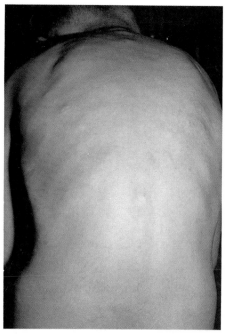

348 Café-au-lait spots in neurofibromatosis, twelve-year-old boy with convulsive disease. His twin brother is also affected by von Recklinghausen's neurofibromatosis.

349 Multiple, faintly visible but well palpable, subcutaneous, neurofibromatous nodules. Histologically: neurofibroma.

Werdnig-Hoffmann Disease *(AUTOS. RECESSIVE)*

Definition

Werdnig-Hoffmann-disease is the infantile form of progressive spinal muscular atrophy. The adult form is called Duchenne-Aran syndrome. The underlying cause of the disease is recessive-hereditary degeneration of anterior horn cells. This results in wasting and pareses of skeletal muscles.

Clinical Findings

Decreased motion is the first sign. It may be noticed in the newborn or sometimes even before birth. Feeble crying and slow feeding follow later. Generalized muscular hypotonia is followed by areflexia and symmetrical flaccid pareses. There will be no progress in static development. Children brought into a sitting position will collapse similar to a pocketknife. Respiration becomes purely abdominal and deficiency of thoracic respiratory muscles causes pigeon-breast deformities of the thorax. Fibrillations are seen on the tongue. Prognosis is hopeless.

↳ DEATH x 2 yrs

Treatment

There is no treatment.

LMN LESION

① ⊖ BABINSKI
② HYPOREFLEXIA
③ F + F
④ FLACCID PARALYSIS
⑤ ABDOM REFLEXES ✓

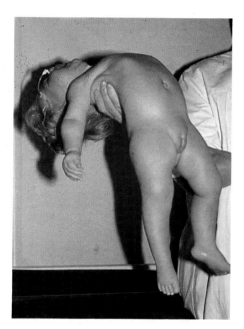

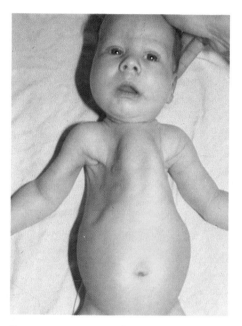

350   Progressive spinal muscular atrophy with severe, generalized muscular hypotonia in a four-month-old infant. Muscular atrophy is concealed by an increased amount of subcutaneous fatty tissue. Three of seven siblings are affected with the disease.

352   Exclusive diaphragmatic respiration with paradoxical respiratory movements. Thoracic deformity caused by paralyzed thoracic respiratory muscles. Death at the age of eight weeks.

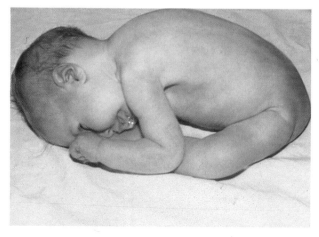

351   Werdnig-Hoffmann disease. Brother of the infant in Fig. 350. Age seven weeks. Pocketknife phenomenon.

Ophthalmic Diseases

Strabismus

Definition

Monocular or alternating internal strabismus is by far the most common form (90 to 95 per cent) of squint during infancy (strabismus convergens). It is due either to hyperopia or to congenital absence of fusion. Strabismus divergens is a rare disorder and generally will not appear before the second decade of life. It may be caused by exophoria, deficient convergence or fusion, or myopia. The general incidence of squint is about four per cent. A familial trait is present in about 40 per cent of the cases.

Clinical Findings

In most cases of monocular squint, the squinting eye shows primary or secondary asthenopia. In alternating convergent squint, neither eye is weak-sighted. The two eyes alternate in occupying the leading role. Uncoordinated ocular motion in the newborn is of no importance (physiologic squint).

Treatment

Strabismus demands treatment by an ophthalmologist early during the second year of life.

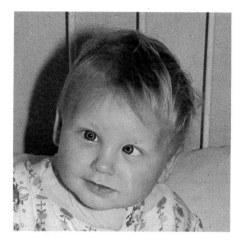

353 Convergent strabismus of the left eye in a 17-month-old boy.

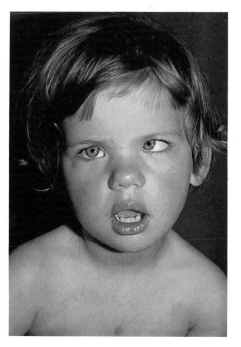 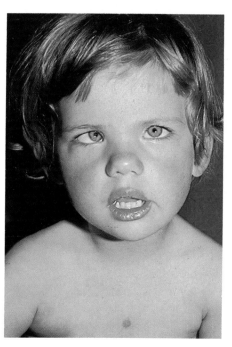

354 and 355 Alternating convergent strabismus in a 30-month-old girl. Familial squinting affliction.

Conjunctivitis

Definition

Conjunctival inflammations may be of exogenous, allergic, or infectious origin. During childhood they are most frequently caused by foreign bodies, pneumococci, staphylococci, streptococci, or viruses. Silver nitrate conjunctivitis, inclusion blenorrhea, and gonococcal blenorrhea are characteristic forms of newborn age.

Clinical Findings

The clinical picture of acute conjunctivitis is characterized by increased lacrimation, reflex closure of eyelids, edematous conjunctiva (chemosis), and serous, hemorrhagic, or purulent secretion.

Treatment

Local treatment depends on etiology, removal of foreign bodies and administration of decongestive agents or antibiotics.

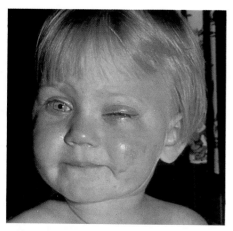

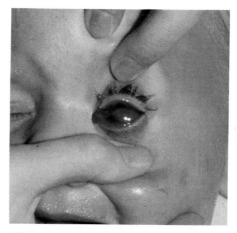

356   Sanguinopurulent conjunctivitis with inflammatory palpebral swelling in a one-year-old girl. No infective agents demonstrated after commencing antibiotic treatment.

357   Eversion of eyelids reveals severe hemorrhagic conjunctival edema (chemosis).

Inflammatory Palpebral Affections

Definition

Local or hematogenous infection by pyogenic agents may cause abscess-forming or phlegmonous inflammation within the loose tissue of eyelids and surrounding soft facial tissue (palpebral abscess, palpebral phlegmon, orbital phlegmon, facial phlegmon). Sty, chalazion, and dacryocystitis caused by stenosis of the tear duct are possible preceding disorders. Inflammatory processes of the facial bones will also cause concomitant palpebral edema. This may indicate osteomyelitis of the upper jaw (odontogenic, maxillary sinusitis), suppurative ethmoiditis, or frontal sinusitis.

Clinical Findings

The primary sign is the closed, swollen eye. In primary infections of the palpebral region, there are striking additional signs of redness, heat, pain and pus at the palpebral fissure. Discreet edema and narrowing of the palpebral fissure are generally the only manifestations of perifocal collateral reactions accompanying deep-lying processes.

Treatment

The principles of therapy consist of internal and local administration of antibiotics, and if necessary, surgical incision.

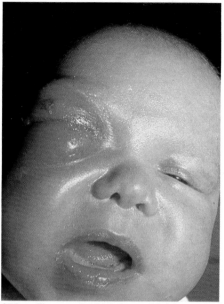

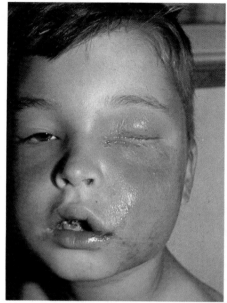

358 Five-week-old infant with abscess of the upper lid. Spontaneous perforation. Staphylococcus aureus haemolyticus was demonstrated. Uneventful healing under combined administration of oxacillin-ampicillin.

359 Phlegmon of the left side of the face in a seven-year-old boy. Orbital soft tissue affected, chemosis and staphylococci in purulent discharge from palpebral fissure. Leukocytes: 20450/µl. Propicillin was an effective treatment.

DACROCYTITIS

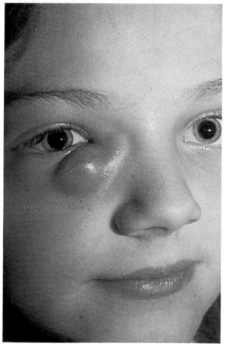

360 Nine-year-old girl with staphylococcal suppuration of the lacrimal sac. Spontaneous perforation occurred on the sixth day of illness. Chloromycetin treatment was curative.

Accidents

Scalding

Definition

Scalding by hot liquids is the most common thermic lesion in infants. If the extent of scalding exceeds 10 per cent of the body surface there are not only local lesions but also signs of shock (primary burn shock).

Clinical Findings

First-degree burns show erythema, second-degree burns vesiculation; healing takes two to three weeks. Third-degree burns are characterized by necroses. Complete healing often takes many weeks.

There is a general rule for estimating the extent of burns: the palmar surface of a child corresponds to about one per cent of the body surface. Apathy, restlessness, pallor with acrocyanosis, and tachycardia are signs of burn shock. Renal failure is a threatening complication. Encephalopathy may remain permanent after burns.

Treatment

Local therapy follows the rules of open-wound treatment. General treatment corresponds to shock therapy.

BODY AREA BURNED

ADULTS
    ↳ Rule of 9'

   · HEAD - 9
    ARMS - 9 x 2.
   · LEGS - 15 x 2
   - TRUNK - 18 x 2
   - PERINEUM - 1%.

CHILD

always expect shock if BSA   >15% ADULTS
                               >10% CHILD.

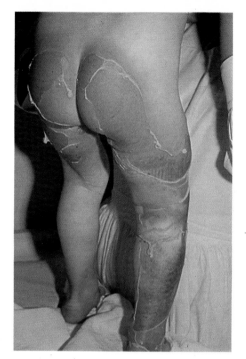

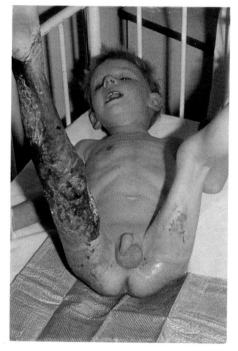

257

361 Second to third-degree scalding of the right leg and buttocks (20 to 25 per cent of body surface affected) after fall into boiling washing solution. Two-year-old boy in shock.

362 Epithelization of second-degree burns after three weeks. Granulation tissue on third-degree burns. Open treatment with antibiotic sprays.

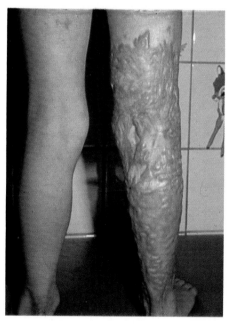

363 Marked keloid formation after 18 months. Flexion contracture of the left knee joint completely eliminated by physiotherapy, full mobility of the joint.

1° DEGREE BURN.
- only epidermis (not derm (outer layer)
- erythema   - tenderness
- ↑ed warmth - pain
- edema.

2° BURN
- damage extends through the epidermis + involves dermis, but not enough to interfere ī rapid regen of epith.
- see vesicles / blebs on bullae.

3° BURN (full thickness)
- both epidermis + dermis are burned.
- nerve endings destroyed

Insect Bites

Definition

Neurotoxic poison of bees, wasps, and ants may cause considerable edema in soft tissue. If the poison enters into the blood stream after venous puncture, central respiratory and circulatory failure may result.

Clinical Findings

Insect bites in the facial area cause Quincke's edema. Swelling in throat and pharynx may cause suffocation.

Treatment

Extraction of the sting, local and intravenous administration of corticosteroids.

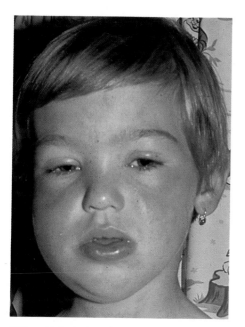

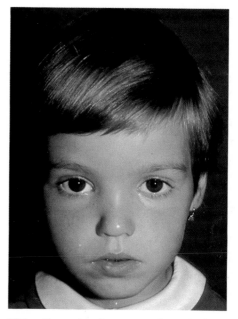

364 Quincke's edema 15 minutes after wasp bite on the right lower lip, in a girl aged 6 years.

365 Normal after two days internal administration of prednisolone.

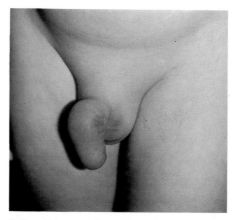

366 Edema of penis with cutaneous hemorrhage caused by gadfly bite. Eliminated by local treatment with cortisone ointment after two days. Age of the boy: three years.

Burns

Definition

In young infants, burns are most frequently caused by hot-water bottles when the temperature of the water exceeds 50° C, when there is no protective wrapping around the bottle, or when an unconscious or an immobilized infant is placed on the bottle. Burns may also be caused by careless application of electric heating pads or lamps.

Clinical Findings

All three degrees of burns are encountered.

261

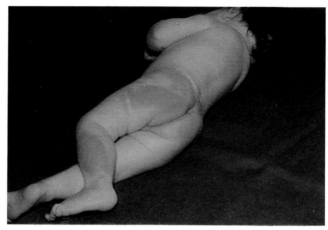

367 First-degree burn by hot-water bottle in a newborn. Cerebral hemorrhage at delivery, hypothermia, and lack of motion were manifestations.

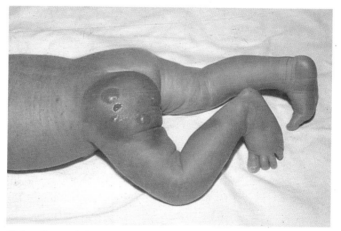

368 Second-degree burn in a newborn caused by a hot-water bottle.

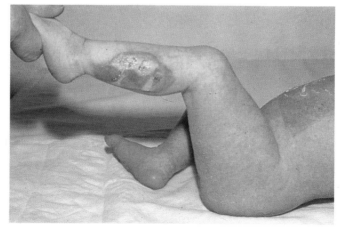

369 Second to third-degree burn by hot-water bottle in a five-week-old infant.

Cranial and Cerebral Injuries

Definition

Within the group of frequent infantile cranial injuries about 50 per cent are soft-tissue injuries, 30 per cent fractures with or without cerebral involvement, and 20 per cent exclusively cerebral injuries. Depending on the degree of severity, the latter may be classified as concussions or contusions.

Clinical Findings

Concussion is characterized by disturbance of consciousness and central vegetative symptoms (vomiting). In contusion additional neurologic focal symptoms are present (convulsions, paralyses, pyramidal signs). In less severe cases they disappear within three weeks, in severe cases symptoms last longer and permanent damage will remain. Uni or bilateral circumocular hematoma may be a manifestation of harmless palpebral contusion or it may be an indication of fractured base of the skull. But, compared to fractures of the cranial convexity, basal fractures are rare during childhood (about ten per cent of all cranial fractures).

Treatment

In concussion, bed rest until spontaneous reactivation will be sufficient. In contusion, additional shock therapy and sedation are required.

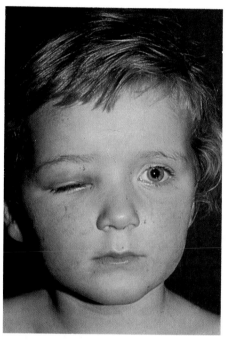

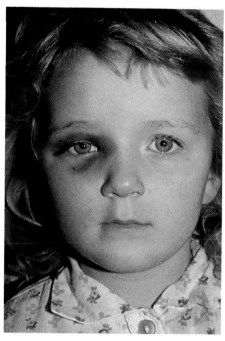

370 A four-year-old girl with bruised eyelid and cerebral concussion after falling down stairs.

371 Swelling of the upper lid has disappeared two days later. In this case, the circumocular hematoma is not an indication that the base of the skull is fractured but of a palpebral contusion.

Pathology Related to Therapy

Facial Petechiae After Gastric Irrigation

Definition

Resistance and straining of a child during gastric irrigation may impair upper venous return causing venous hyperemia and capillary diapedetic hemorrhage in the facial area. This corresponds to Rumpel-Leede phenomenon.

Clinical Findings

Petechial hemorrhage of facial skin and conjunctivae.

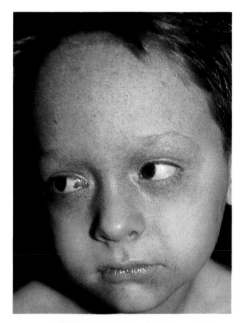

372   Facial and conjunctival hemorrhage caused by gastric irrigation because of accidental ingestion of alcohol; boy five years, seven months.

Exanthematous Drug Reactions

Definition

During childhood a great variety of drug allergies may appear. A number of drugs may cause allergic cutaneous reactions: above all penicillin derivatives, barbiturates, analgesics, and antiepileptic drugs. In primary sensitization, the lesions often appear around the ninth day (fourth to 20th day) after intake of the allergen. There is no correlation between different manifestations and different drugs.

Clinical Findings

All types of exanthem may be met with: erythematous, scarlatiniform, rubelliform, morbilliform, urticarial, papulous (strophulus), infiltrating (erythema nodosum), vesicular, acneiform, and hemorrhagic changes of the skin. The picture of erythema exudativum multiforme may be present (See p. 218) or the severe manifestations of epidermolysis acuta toxica (Lyell's syndrome).

Differential Diagnosis

Differentiation of exanthematous infectious disease is based upon history (verification of allergen), epidemiology, and course of the disease. Often, exanthematous drug reactions do not produce systemic disturbances.

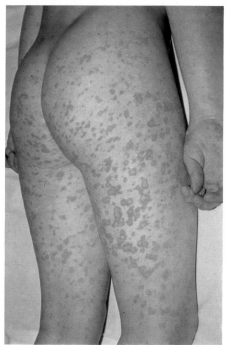

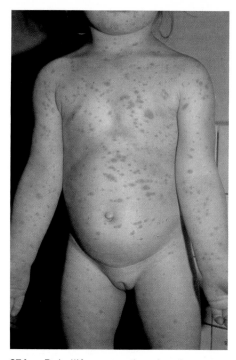

373 Morbilliform-urticarial drug eruption nine days after intramuscular administration of ampicillin, ten-year-old girl. Deflorescence after five days.

374 Rubelliform exanthem in a three-year-old girl, nine days after oral administration of ampicillin.

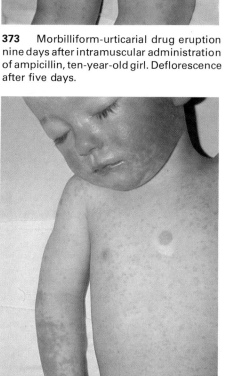

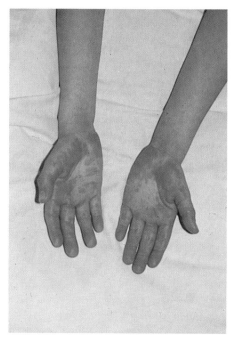

375 Phenobarbital exanthem one week after rectal administration: rubelliform eruptions on the trunk, morbilliform-confluent eruptions on the lower arm, diffuse erythema in face.

376 Palmar erythema may be the manifestation of a drug reaction, as shown here; it may appear in cirrhosis of the liver or in vegetative lability.

Atrophic Cutaneous Striae

Definition

Striae distensae is the Latin name for striae caused by distended skin which only appears in children and young adults. An increased plasma level of glucocorticosteroids (systemic administration of corticosteroids, Cushing's disease, pregnancy) causes damage of elastic fibers manifested by cutaneous striae.

Clinical Findings

Reversible striae appear on abdomen and thighs. In the beginning they show a bluish-red color, later that of mother-of-pearl.

Gingival Hyperplasia

[handwritten annotations: → anti-epileptic meds; → acute myeloses; → tuberous scleroses; → cyanotic heart disease; → idiopathic gingival fibromatosis — hypertrichosis, — cranial deform., — cranial deform., — gynecomastia]

Definition

Fibromatous gingival hyperplasia may be a side effect to antiepileptic hydantoin therapy, to acute myeloses (10 per cent), tuberous sclerosis, and cyanotic heart disease. Dominant, hereditary, idiopathic gingival fibromatosis is a rare disorder combined with hypertrichosis, cranial deformities, and gynecomastia.

Clinical Findings

Painless, cosmetically disturbing overgrowth of gingival margins. With poor oral hygiene, the disorder facilitates the development of gingivitis.

Treatment

Possibly surgical excision. Oral hygiene.

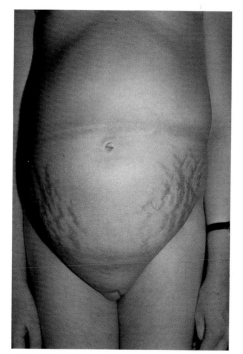

377 Formation of striae caused by nephrotic syndrome in an eleven-year-old girl after five months of continuous prednisolone administration (methyl-prednisolone).

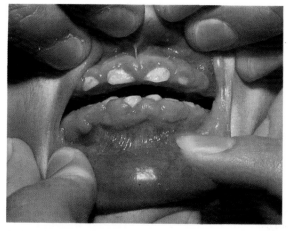

378 Gingival hyperplasia on the lower jaw after mephenytoin treatment.

Index